The Nell Dialogues

The Nell Dialogues

Conversation in Mortal Time

RICHARD P. MCQUELLON, PHD

Comprehensive Cancer Center
Wake Forest Baptist Health, NC, USA

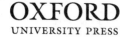

OXFORD
UNIVERSITY PRESS

OXFORD

UNIVERSITY PRESS

Oxford University Press is a department of the University of Oxford. It furthers
the University's objective of excellence in research, scholarship, and education
by publishing worldwide. Oxford is a registered trade mark of Oxford University
Press in the UK and certain other countries.

Published in the United States of America by Oxford University Press
198 Madison Avenue, New York, NY 10016, United States of America.

Library of Congress Cataloging-in-Publication Data
Names: McQuellon, Richard P., 1949- interviewer, editor.
Title: The Nell dialogues : conversation in mortal time /
Richard McQuellon, editor.
Description: New York, NY : Oxford University Press, [2022] |
Includes bibliographical references and index.
Identifiers: LCCN 2021023848 (print) | LCCN 2021023849 (ebook) |
ISBN 9780190091019 (paperback) | ISBN 9780190091033 (epub) |
ISBN 9780190091040 (ebook)
Subjects: MESH: Neoplasms—psychology | Patients—psychology |
Attitude to Death | Attitude to Health | Quality of Life |
Terminal Care—psychology | Interview
Classification: LCC RC271.M4 (print) | LCC RC271.M4 (ebook) | NLM QZ 260 |
DDC 616.99/40651—dc23
LC record available at https://lccn.loc.gov/2021023848
LC ebook record available at https://lccn.loc.gov/2021023849

DOI: 10.1093/med/9780190091019.001.0001

1 3 5 7 9 8 6 4 2

Printed by Marquis, Canada

This book is dedicated to Nell and Al M., who opened their hearts and home to me in their final days of grief and celebration in mortal time.

Contents

Preface

We die with the dying:
See, they depart, and we go with them.
We are born with the dead:
See, they return, and bring us with them.

T.S. Eliot, *Little Gidding*

The pages of this book are windows on a remarkable conversation between a person responding to dying by living more fully and the psychotherapist accompanying her in that profound aspiration. *The Nell Dialogues* offer a rare invitation for readers to witness a sustained conversation in mortal time, those moments when human beings confront death personally or vicariously.

Authentic communication is never controlled by the agenda of either party. It raises questions for both. We encounter the personal questioning arising from genuine dialogue in these moving conversations. Nell wonders what awaits her in dying and beyond. Her psychotherapist agonizes over whether the ethics of his profession are constraining him unnecessarily from meeting her more fully in her time of departing.

If Nell's raw honesty leaves readers squirming at times, her intelligence, humor, and tenacity are edifying. Her spiritual curiosity about the nature of reality ceases (or is transformed) only in her dying. The soul-searching of her conversation partner, whose remarkable and hazardous vocation has been to be a consoling presence to the dying and their loved ones in a comprehensive cancer care center, will evoke empathetic recognition in anyone who engages seriously with the dying, their families, or anyone in life-threatening pain, whether physical or psychological.

The mystical philosopher Martin Buber wrote: "The basis of our lives together is two-fold and it is one—the wish of every person to be confirmed by others as what they are and what they can become; and our innate capacity to confirm one another in this way." In the conversation between Nell and her companion, the mutual acknowledgment that is truly "the basis our lives together," but usually goes unremarked, emerges into visibility for a sacred moment, offering readers a glimpse of the relational depths of the present and of the time awaiting us all in the future.

The dying depart, and we go with them.

Michael A. Cowan
Professor Emeritus,
Loyola University New Orleans
Centre for the Study of Social Cohesion,
University of Oxford

Acknowledgments

The Nell Dialogues: Conversation in Mortal Time

Writing this book was challenging. It stirred the grief that was my companion during my time with Nell. The echoes of that grief returned as our story was relived in the writing. This book fulfills the promise I made to Nell. I could not have written it without the help of the people named here. Many have been with me over the course of my professional career in cancer medicine.

To Dr. Michael Cowan, my loyal friend and colleague of 58 years, my heartfelt thank you. Mike recognized the need for commentary interspersed in our dialogues to provide a window into the therapist's thinking and feeling. I am deeply grateful for his insight. Our story is the better for it. Mike's friendship has passed the endurance test for sure, supporting me over three decades in mortal time.

I am grateful to my teaching colleague, Wake Forest University Professor Emerita of English, Women's, Gender and Sexuality studies Dr. Mary DeShazer, for her generous, diligent reading and rereading of this manuscript. Her detailed editing and suggestions were invaluable, adding to coherence and readability. Her role as co-director of our Pro Humanitate program for Wake Forest University students and steady companionship in our hematology/oncology clinic provided energy to help complete the task. Her success teaching me the correct use of possessive nouns is a testament to her patience.

Dr. Dennis O'Hara has been my steadfast friend and colleague since 1978. During the period I worked with and wrote about Nell, he was a constant source of encouragement. His careful listening and wise counsel over the years as well as thoughtful feedback on an earlier version of this manuscript has made the difference, helping to sustain me in cancer care. Dennis knows the heartbreak of accompanying a loved one at the end of life.

A special thanks to psychologist and priest Dr. Richard Chiles, a wise clinical supervisor. He taught the importance of deep listening. There is always another layer to the person, a deeper story to understand. After the words are spoken, the dialogue continues to be analyzed in the mind and heart of the listening therapist.

I owe a debt of gratitude to our section chief of Hematology and Oncology, Dr. Bayard Powell, and our Wake Forest Baptist Medical Center, Comprehensive Cancer Center director, Dr. Boris Pasche. Their constant care of the Cancer Patient Support Program (CPSP) allowed me the time to write Nell's story.

I was fortunate to find a wise medical mentor early in my career. I will always be grateful to Dr. Hy Muss, who taught that patients can manage metastatic disease and that hope can be communicated in a smile and a hug.

Thank you to:

- My coworkers in the Cancer Patient Support Program. Gail Hurt provided unwavering accompaniment on the journey with Nell as well as poems by Mary Oliver. Gail was my guide in the darkness. Sheila Lee carefully typed the first version of the transcripts while at the same time organizing the work of the CPSP. Pat Dechatelet, who directed our volunteers, and Suzanne Danhauer, who shared the clinical care of patients; I am fortunate to have regular companions in mortal time, Dr. Katie Duckworth, Andrea Edwards, Stephanie Lichiello, Dr. Ruth Moskop, Victoria O'Connor, Dr. Lisa Rainwater, and Aimee Tolbert, my current coworkers in the CPSP.
- My nurse and physician colleagues in medicine and medical, surgical, and radiation oncology who taught me how to see

the biological in the biopsychosocial model of medical care: Drs. Mebs Aklilu, Katharine Ansley, Angela Alistair, Christine Bishop, William Blackstock, Dale Browne, Tom Dubose, Julia Cruz, Leslie Ellis, Andrew Farland, Carolyn Ferree, Stefan Grant, Carl Grey, Diana Howard, David Hurd, Heidi Klepin, Glenn Lesser, Denise Levitan, Ed Levine, Thomas Lycan, Nelson May, Michael McCormack, Christopher Miles, Tony Miller, Richard Patterson, Jeff Petty, Perry Shen, Caio Rocha Lima, Paul Savage, Mary Beth Seegars, Steve Sorscher, Alexandra Thomas, Chris Thomas, and George Yacoub; Susan Lyerly, PA-C, Rebecca Murray, PA-C, Nathan Ogilvie, PA-C and Kate Winterbottom, MS, CCC-SLP; Nurses Makia Cade, Sally Cowgill, Terena Reese, Jennifer Woodberry, Abby Laurence.

- Our fellowship director, Dr. Susan Melin and the exceptional Hematology/Oncology fellows who discussed difficult patient encounters in cancer medicine, and especially Dr. Gabe McCoy, whose essay on purpose informs the concept of resilience.
- Dr. Ed Starin, who believed in me and the promise of psychosocial care of patients, and Dr. K. Patrick Ober for his humor, insight, and wisdom.
- Internal Medicine Department Chairs Drs. Bill Hazard, Bill Applegate, Tom Debose, and Gary Rosenthal.
- The Wake Forest Comprehensive Cancer Center and Hematology/Oncology administrators, the people behind the scenes who hold our work together: Janet Forest, Debbie Olson, Tina Martin, Donna Pranke, Rebecca Rankin, Valar Wilson, and Holly Amazon.
- Amy Peterman, director of clinical training at University of North Carolina Charlotte, for sending curious, dedicated, and diligent students to learn in the trying setting of surgical oncology and especially practicum student Olivia Riffle, companion with laryngectomy patients and author of *Learning the Language of Silence*.

- Marian and Jimmy Douglas, Ann and Borden Hanes, and Lynn and Jeff Young, who have supported me and the CPSP over the decades.

I appreciate the following groups, who provide both the human and material resources to sustain our cancer patient support program:

- The Wake Forest University undergraduate Pro Humanitate students who brought life and energy to the CPSP and especially to Dr. Jared Rejeski, who was our first Pro Humanitate intern, leading the way with diligence and compassion.
- CPSP volunteers, whose loyal care of patients is a source of healing in our clinics: Agnes Barry, Skip Boyles, Sam Bright, Tom Chadwick, Judy Ditmore, Doris Dick, Rose Dubose, Dr. Ed Easley, Ronnie Flowers, Linda Gitter, Ernestine Glenn, Jerry Gray, Hermine and Bob Heller, Kathy Janeway, Roger Jordan, Ray Joyner, Martha Kinney, Trinette Kirkman, Noreen Lee, Joyce and Jim Lindberg, Bertha Long, May Merleau, Cathy Mills, Kris Morris, Tatiana Oborskaya, Cynthia Robertson, Vicki Selner, and Jim and Pat Stoeber.
- The courageous nurses, physicians, residents, and fellows on the otolaryngology and surgical oncology services, who encounter some of the most heartbreaking and difficult medical situations in cancer care.
- Healing musicians: Our Lady of Mercy choir and director Dr. Diane Caruso, the source of energy holding us together for over 20 years. Singing in the choir has been a soothing elixir for the suffering felt in cancer medicine; The Healing Harps for their restorative music in our cancer center; the Shades of Praise New Orleans Interracial Gospel Choir, whose songs of praise are magic, uplifting patients with titles such as "My Healing." The Shade of praise lifted me up.

- The office of Philanthropy and Alumni Affairs, and especially Carolyn Beckman, Allison Brouillette, Cindy Caines, Susan Kennedy, Lisa Marshall, Jennifer Woodward, and all the Winterlark fundraiser chairs and volunteers who helped sustain our CPSP.

I am grateful for the wisdom and advice of professional colleagues Drs. Mike Andrykowski, Teresa Deshields, Paul Fox, and Shannon Nana, and to Cassie Campbell, Lib Edwards, Greg Kucera, Anna Lehman, Loretta Muss, Tim Rambo, Greg Russell, and companions on the road in cancer medicine. Dr. Pat Lustman and Dr. Claudia Sowa, fellow Michigan State University Spartans, whose presence during and after graduate school has been source of energy for the task of writing. Healing conversation with my colleagues has been a source of renewal over the years.

I am grateful for my special community of friends who have sustained my spirits in the dark times: Pat and Ed Hamlin, David and Madeline Harold, Jim and Rosemary Irion, Barry and Sandra Maine, Mark Rabil, Sue and Phillipe Sevin.

I appreciate my editors and readers: author and Wake Forest University English Department faculty member Julie Edelson, who made first edits; Amber Alsobrooks, who read and provided helpful insights and editorial suggestions early, helping shape the narrative. Thanks to everyone on the Oxford University Press team: Jacqueline Buckley, Sujitha Logaganesan, and especially managing editor Andrea Knobloch, who encouraged me to tell Nell's story. The talent of graphic artist Alice Sanders is visible on the cover. I thank her for patience with the author.

To my patients, who have taught me what it means to hold steady in the deepening shade of mortal time. They are woven into the heart of these dialogues.

- To my family, Meghan and Dr. Greg, Dillon and Bowen McCandless; Dr. Brendan McQuellon, Kelly and Evelyn Ruth. Your presence has given purpose and deep meaning all these years. The call of mortality is quiet in your company.
- My wife, Cyndee, read every page and lived through my journey with Nell. She shared the painful and triumphant moments of Nell's story as it was lived and relived in the writing. Her steady presence eased the inevitable suffering set loose in the company of loss. Nell's story reawakened my own sorrow, the companion of conversation in mortal time. Your Love is a powerful, life-sustaining force, making all the difference. I will always be grateful. What better companion on earth.

Richard P. McQuellon

Introduction

The Prospect of Mortality

The problem is despair. I don't know how I can go on.

Nell M.

This book tells the story of Nell M., a 61-year-old writer and art historian diagnosed on December 31, 2003, with metastatic breast cancer. It presents 12 of our dialogues from February 16, 2005, until her death on June 22, 2005, with my commentaries. Our therapeutic relationship began in September 2004 as biweekly sessions at Wake Forest Baptist Health (WFBH), where I have worked for 30 years as a psychosocial oncologist. As Nell became increasingly aware of her death on the near horizon, we began to record our meetings, initially at the medical center, then in her home.

The primary purpose of this illness narrative is to illustrate one brave woman's encounter with *mortal time*, by which I mean the heightened awareness and experience of our own mortality. I also offer a window on the world of patients and their caregivers facing life-threatening illness together. As Nell's story unfolded, it became a story about our relationship as well. These dialogues trace Nell's acceptance of, and struggle with, the practical obstacles to achieving a good death.

To believe in this living is just a hard way to go.

John Prine, "Angel from Montgomery"

After five months of chemotherapy, when, in her words, "our treatments failed, and the tumor went galloping free all the way across my torso," Nell decided to stop treatment. Her medical oncologist informed her that "we are in the months range now." Several months later, when her expected expiration date had passed, she came to see me on the recommendation of her friend, a fellow patient with breast cancer I knew. She was depressed and despairing. She had seen her limited lifespan as a reprieve from watching the brilliant mind of her spouse, Al, deteriorate due to Alzheimer's disease. Now she was still on earth, bracing for her worst fear: his long, slow decline toward death. Later in our conversations, she gained a new perspective, accepting Al's illness and what it meant for them both as an opportunity to deal with previous problems in their relationship.

I had never heard any cancer patient describe extended life as a disappointment. Nell thought she had only months to live, yet she was very much alive and frustrated that her expected death date had come and gone. How did she come to see her dismal breast cancer prognosis as a welcome ticket out of this world? When she spoke of her beloved spouse's Alzheimer's disease, I began to understand the imagined future she wanted to avoid and breast cancer as her exit strategy. She also feared life without Al. We entered into this territory, familiar to me as a long-time professional resident of Cancerland,[1] a place that regularly prompts the question about how patients manage in mortal time.

This question was the central focus of an article I wrote with my colleague Michael Cowan, "Turning Toward Death Together: Conversation in Mortal Time."[2] It was our first effort to make sense of how cancer patients can live with death as an all-too-real prospect. I encountered "mortal time" in an essay titled "One Night's Dying" by anthropologist and mystical naturalist Loren Eiseley.[3] He used it to describe the stark finality of our brief existence. We wanted to illuminate this challenge facing cancer patients, one that Nell engaged with great courage. I gave the article to Nell because I thought its title would stimulate her curiosity, rather than fear. She appreciated it because it spoke to her situation. It was an invitation to address her own mortality in the safety of our conversations.

Who Was Nell?

Nell G. M. was born in 1944 and grew up in a small town south of Pittsburgh, which she loved for the diversity of its population and the beauty of its setting. She had two sisters, Ruth and Joyce, and two brothers, John and Walter.

She graduated from Wheaton College in 1966 with a degree in English literature and French and worked as a writer and editor in Chicago with Studs Terkel on his massive project *Working: People Talk About What They Do All Day and How They Feel About What They Do*.

In 1974, she moved to Washington, DC, and began collecting primitive American folk art and furniture. In 1976, she moved to New York City, where, in 1978, she opened an art gallery exploring the relationships among several genres. She became increasingly interested in the history of religions and the history of art, which drew her to earn a Master of Arts degree in religion from Columbia University in 1984. In the same year, she married Al, a retired Columbia University professor of religion.

The couple moved to North Carolina when Al accepted a position as a professor at Wake Forest University in Winston-Salem. Nell entered the University of North Carolina (UNC) at Chapel Hill and studied art history, receiving a Master of Arts in 1988 and a PhD in 1995. Her area of expertise was the illustration of 12th- and 13th-century devotional literature in England and France. Over the course of her teaching career, she held appointments at Duke University, UNC Chapel Hill, and North Carolina School of the Arts. However, she would later say that she was most gratified when teaching eighth-grade language arts and social studies at Hill Magnet School for the Performing and Visual Arts in Winston-Salem.

Nell loved nature. When she and Al sold their home and moved into an apartment because of declining health, she gave up her flower garden and some of her prized artwork and furniture. She could still set her bird feeders on the balcony. She filled them religiously and sat for hours watching cardinals, finches, and chickadees and clouds massing on the horizon.

The transcribed dialogues that follow developed out of a trusting relationship and growing mutual respect and reverence for conversation and its power to illuminate mortal time. We did not begin therapy with the idea of recording our conversations; however, it became clear that Nell had lessons to teach the dying and the living. As a person of letters and a writer, she naturally wanted to share her reflections with others encountering mortal time as a guide to a good ending.

In his essay "A Good Death: Exit Strategies," William Vollmann states, "There must be better and worse ways to die. It seems both rational and possible to minimize the likelihood of an unpleasant end. What then about a 'good death'? Is such a thing possible?"[4] At first, Nell considered her diagnosis a parachute that would spare her the suffering attendant on the slow deterioration of her spouse's sharp intellect and her angst about a future without him. Eventually, however, she changed and began to seek a good death for herself while Al could still recognize her. He was already becoming withdrawn and more forgetful; he was losing his remarkable ability to recall facts from his academic work in religion and philosophy. In our therapy sessions, Nell worked to accept his illness and her loss of his intellectual companionship, which allowed her to find meaning in her own suffering and a renewed sense of purpose. She stopped hoping for a quick exit and started hoping to create a good life and death in her expanded mortal time. She was choosing a different path than the one her breast cancer had initiated.

Nell often paraphrased the first lines of "Verses on the Faith Mind" by Chien-chih Seng-ts'an, Third Patriarch of Zen (606 AD).[5] The poem begins, "The great way is not difficult for those with no preferences." She often said, "The great way is not difficult if you just don't pick and choose." She realized that our culture has spawned an advertising industry designed to shape consumer preferences, to convince people what to choose to buy each day. She was trying to accept her situation and roll with the everyday tasks of living in mortal time, yet she struggled with her own preferences for her last days.

Of course, unless you are a monk, sequestered away from the everyday demands of life, making choices is what we must do each day. How could this responsibility be less salient at the end of life for someone like Nell? Each day, she had to navigate her bodily needs: to adjust her nasal cannula just right so she would get oxygen, to fill the oxygen filter with water to prevent her nasal passages from drying out, to calculate how much energy she might have to meet and greet various visitors. These daily choices became poignant with the end horizon in sight. It initiated a spiritual search.

The Role of Spirituality and Prayer

Nell was an intensely spiritual person, and her Catholic Christian faith and Buddhist leanings informed much of our conversation/interactions. She was not a literalist, yet she valued the Bible and referred to it frequently. The spiritual dimension of our work together is best reflected by this quote from Dr. Daniel Sulmasy: "The primary spiritual act is the expression of empathic concern."[6] I understand this phrase to mean *loving is listening* since the primary spiritual act is to love one another. Intense listening was characteristic of our conversation throughout. Late in our relationship, when she was bedridden, Nell would ask to me to say a prayer at the end of our meetings, which I did as we both shared the same faith tradition. Something about the vulnerability of her position called for a message to the transcendent. We were reaching for the heavens in these moments.

Nell was, in her words, "a fitfully practicing Catholic," and had explored Buddhism and adopted meditative practices. She appreciated the Buddhist perspective on suffering. She saw that it studies suffering in all its forms: what they are, and how they may be transformed in a way of living that minimizes suffering. She strived to understand her own suffering without focusing on herself except to give meaning to the attitudes and behavior related to her suffering. She sought self-transformation and self-improvement by managing and intentionally embracing her illness.

Toward the end, she became more aware of the need to die well with the help of her own faith tradition. Consequently, she enlisted her parish priests and lay workers from her church. Her priests would visit and offer prayers. She received the Sacrament of the Anointing of the Sick. A parish volunteer who visited regularly and prayed with her hooked up her TV so she could watch the Tennis Channel's nonstop coverage of her passion. The rhythmic movement and competitive shouts from the tennis stars gave her respite from the daily background buzz of mortal time.

The Structure of This Book

Nell edited our first four conversations in an effort to draw out what she wanted to teach. She did only minor edits on additional dialogues and read a total of nine; she came to see our work as a developmental sequence in facing, accepting, and yielding to death. In the last weeks, her energy began to wane, and she was increasingly focused on the day-to-day realities of living in a withering body.

I have edited the original transcribed dialogues and drawn from Nell's revised versions, remaining true to the exchange and yet amplifying her voice to illustrate what she wanted to convey. In some cases, this gives more scope to Nell's own narrative and leaves our verbal exchange in the background. The nonverbal exchanges that accompany these dialogues, while not visible to the reader, were critical to our conversation. Our actions, including occasionally holding hands near the end, and particularly facial cues that conveyed empathy, encouragement, and reassurance, were essential components of our interaction. It is impossible to convey all such gestures well in a written dialogue. During many conversations, there were especially poignant wordless exchanges and pauses, which are shown, to some extent, in the pages that follow.

Recording gave new energy to our conversations. Given Nell's expertise in writing and editing, she found satisfaction in telling, recording, and making meaning of the last phase of her story. I had some misgivings before asking her to record, as I did not want the process to get in the way of our therapeutic relationship. Rather than being an obstacle, however, the recording seemed to enhance our work by adding the prospect that the words would live on for others engaging mortal time. Nell found the process of reading and editing the dialogues helpful and meaningful. Reading quieted her mind to the background buzz of mortality, which she said was always there. I have woven her changes into our dialogues in a way that keeps the story whole.

Sheila Lee, administrative assistant for the Cancer Patient Support Program, transcribed all of the recorded sessions. If she was uncertain about a word or phrase, we would listen to the tape together to ensure accuracy. I would then review the transcribed dialogue and make additional corrections as needed.

I emailed the transcribed dialogues to Nell, and she edited them to highlight certain poignant exchanges before returning them to me. We often discussed recurrent themes and other salient points, as in any therapy. Reading her own words stimulated Nell.

The book represents 14 meetings and 12 recorded conversations that took place over a period of 17 weeks. While each conversation is separate, a continuous thread runs through them: themes of managing physically, psychologically, socially, and spiritually at life's end. When we met the day before Nell died, there was no recording. The evening she died, I sat at her bedside with her spouse Al and the hospice nurse in the next room. I discuss those meetings in Chapter 13.

Each of these meetings began with some conversation among Al, Nell, and me. The topic would be the news of the day or Al's activities and would include an offer of something to drink. He would talk for bit and then leave us to speak privately. At the end of each session, we scheduled our next meeting and I responded to any questions Nell had. In our final several meetings, we read a poem or prayed together at her invitation. I omitted the beginning and end of some of the dialogues to provide the most useful content to the reader.

Coping with Cancer, Symptoms, Relationships, Thoughts, Feelings and Role Changes

All patients diagnosed with cancer are challenged to cope with stressors in four major areas that overlap and affect one another. They are always in the background and more or less present in each of our exchanges. The dialogues with Nell illustrate these areas of concern.

Disease and symptoms are the first stressor. Coping well is dependent on understanding the nature of the cancer diagnosis, learning about treatment alternatives, and making choices when the best path forward is uncertain. Both the disease and its treatment cause a variety of symptoms, including fatigue, pain, nausea, and lack of energy. Managing them calls for clear and open communication with healthcare providers, who usually know of solutions. It also requires some familiarity with how our own bodies work.

How do I make sense of how my body is responding? Do I have a low or high tolerance for pain and nausea? What does this pain mean? Is it "normal" for chemotherapy? Should I call my doctor about the numbness in my toes? Patients vary dramatically in their awareness of how their body works and are more or less able to analyze their situation and decide what might be helpful. All other things being equal, people with a history of managing symptoms will be better able to help their medical provider to understand and know what to do with the symptoms they encounter due to cancer or its treatment. People who are accustomed to keeping bodily discomfort and even pain to themselves may find it difficult to articulate a symptom so that the treatment team can be helpful. Some patients have to learn what different bodily sensations mean to know when to sound the alarm and when to let it be. When to call on the treatment team is a key task in effective disease and symptom management.

Over time, lack of energy and low endurance became more of a problem for Nell. They were a product of her changing nutritional status, low hemoglobin, sleep disruption as well as increased time in bed, pain medication, and the progression of her disease. Effective use of oxygen, varying her diet, and a blood transfusion helped her to regain energy and a sense of vitality in her last weeks. Pain at the site of her expanding tumor was also a companion toward the end. Nell became adept at reporting her needs to her medical team, a difficult task at times, as you will learn.

Personal and professional relationships are the second area of potential difficulty. Relationships with family and friends invariably change over the course of cancer treatment, for better and worse. Some people become closer while others fall away. In Nell's case, she was navigating the difficult cancer diagnosis and treatment course, while Al's Alzheimer's disease was changing their relationship at a time when she needed his emotional support and care. It also underscored the intermittent nature of their emotional closeness over the years at a time when Nell craved deep connection, which she enhanced over time with Al and her family.

Nell utilized and valued home hospice help after a rocky start with them while still under the care of her kind, competent medical oncologist, who had been following her for many months. Phone calls and sensitive conversations with the principal people from each group were required. In the dialogues, Nell identifies problems with her professional caregivers and the need to repeat herself and clarify problems in order to solve them. She also speaks of difficult but necessary changes in her friendship network as she became more homebound with less dexterity and energy.

Thoughts and feelings are the third area. Intrusive thoughts in the form of repeated self talk about threats to physical well-being can be debilitating. For example, the thought "This chemotherapy is killing me" is discouraging and self-defeating. It intrudes on and can erode life's quality. Fear of recurrence, progressive disease or debilitating symptoms are troubling. Nell feared she would experience a terrifying sense of suffocation as she died. Such a disturbing thought of a painful death can create incapacitating feelings of anxiety, sadness, depression, hopelessness, and helplessness.

Many psychological techniques are useful for reducing the debilitating anxiety that fuels intrusive thoughts. They include guided imagery, mindfulness-based stress reduction, and simple breathing techniques. The tenacity of psychological symptoms is illustrated by cancer survivor and poet Ted Kooser when he likens anxiety to the "daredevil squirrel of worry" who cannot be quieted by the recommended baffles, "tin cone of meditation, greased pipe of positive thought."[7] Nell used guided imagery, breathing techniques, and antianxiety medication to help settle herself when panic about swallowing engulfed her. She reported gaining mastery over her feelings by talking about them and analyzing them in our conversations.

Finally, *valued life roles and tasks* in life may vary dramatically during and following cancer treatment. Work and leisure activities necessarily change with the waxing and waning of physical symptoms. Patients often refer to the "roller coaster" ride of being a patient with uncertainty being the only predictable course forward. As Nell's condition deteriorated and mobility was limited she had to give up many roles and activities such as cooking, meetings with friends, dinners out with Al and importantly, church attendance.

Therapeutic Approach and Process

The counseling approach in our meetings could best be described as supportive-expressive psychotherapy (SEP) along with problem-solving. SEP is a time-limited, focused psychotherapy that has two main components: supportive techniques, such as empathic listening, and expressive techniques, such as encouraging patients to identify and work through interpersonal relationship problems.[8] This approach has been used in group therapy, where psychological distress in patients with metastatic breast cancer was managed successfully.[9]

These techniques facilitated the development of a trusting relationship where Nell could express her deepest fears and disappointments. Listening carefully and responding thoughtfully were the crucible of healing since they can activate an empathic connection. Throughout our conversations, Nell worked to understand the meaning of her living and dying experience. Expressing her emotions, putting her feelings into words, had therapeutic benefit for her. According to Egan, from a psychological standpoint, these benefits include clarifying the problem situation, reducing anxiety, evolving an action plan, and increasing a sense of self-efficacy.[10] Research in the neurosciences has shown that labeling our emotions has differential effects on specific areas of the brain: The amygdala is less active, and the right ventrolateral prefrontal cortex is more active. When people put feelings into words, they may lessen unpleasant responses.[11] Talking about how we feel has beneficial effects both psychologically and physiologically.

Empathic *listening* is communicated through nonverbal cues from eyes and face, voice tone, and silence. Listening is deceptively powerful in affirming the other and inviting further self-revelation in the service of action and/or self-soothing.[12]

For the most part, our problem-solving focused on symptom management. At one point, Nell had to talk with hospice phone operators and nurses to ensure that her pain medication would be ordered and arrive on time. Frequently, interpersonal issues and intrusive thoughts troubled her over the course of our meetings and required rational analysis and ideas about how to change them. You will also see elements of the well-regarded dignity therapy— maintaining autonomy and control—in our conversations.[13]

Our therapeutic alliance and affective bond developed quickly and formed the foundation of our work together. Initially, our relationship was enhanced by our shared interest in the concept of mortal time and the credibility Nell assigned me based on my relationship with her friend Linda, a breast cancer patient I had seen and come to know as a professional colleague. Nell wanted to understand the meaning of her living and dying process. In our first several meetings, we came to an agreement about the primary goal and process of therapy. Our broad goal of negotiating a course toward a good death, evolved over time and included addressing old difficulties in Nell's marriage and family of origin that emerged after thoroughly discussing her feeling of despair. Nell felt Al was emotionally distant, and she needed him now. You will see in these dialogues her dawning awareness of the tasks to be done in her living–dying interval.

I have attempted to illustrate the therapeutic process more clearly by commenting on the dialogue. The commentary is designed to unpack the discipline while noting the spontaneity of our conversation in a variation of what Professor Norman

Kagan described as *interpersonal process recall*, where the therapist reviews a video of the session and stops the tape occasionally
to comment on the interpersonal process.[14,15] The discipline that
should tell the therapist when to speak and when to remain silent
is a product of professional training and experience. However,
therapists who continually and systematically track themselves
and analyze every utterance risk becoming reductionist clinician
robots. Spontaneity in conversation gives counseling life. The
hallmark of good therapeutic engagement involves both discipline and spontaneity. Inviting and often leading the conversation
with a willing patient partner are the therapist's responsibility.

The dialogues are informed by nature, poetry, music, and, to
some extent, consoling touch. Nell was comforted by the wind, sun,
and birds visible from her apartment balcony and windows. Mary
Oliver's poems speak to Nell's love of nature as well as her encounter
with death. With regard to music, toward the end, she played *Rosa
Mystica* every night, in which gifted musician and mystic Therese
Schroeder-Sheker's pure soprano voice and harp accompaniments
weave a cocoon of care around the listener. Schroeder-Sheker plays
ancient Irish, Romanian, Israeli, and Sephardic melodies on the
album with a beauty and clarity that transcend time. Nell fell asleep
in the company of the melodic music with Al at her bedside. During
our meetings, she would often reach to hold my hand for comfort
and a solid connection to the world of the living. While I have not
been trained in healing touch, a form of energy healing available
at our institution,[16] Nell found the occasional gesture of consoling
touch helpful and healing.

Many people walked with Nell during her mortal time experience. I have changed the names of her professional caregivers as
well as the priests and laypeople from her church. The first names of
her family members and closest friends remain. Even though Nell
gave permission to use her full name, I have omitted it to protect
the privacy of her family.

The Art of Dying

In the pages that follow, I am the listening partner in an intense dialogue. I address the reader with reflective/interpretive commentary on the highlights and subtleties. Each meeting is introduced with an orienting reflection, where I summarize themes and set up an expectation of what is coming for the reader. The text is two-dimensional: the dialogue and my thoughts and feelings as the privileged participant-observer and Nell's intimate companion in mortal time. The commentary provides me with a unique opportunity to shed compassionate light on her living in mortal time. I end the book with reflections on entering mortal time with Nell.

This book is a contribution to the literature of *Ars moriendi*, the art of dying.[17] Narratives illustrating what Dr. Atul Gawande has called "being mortal" in ways that can be lifegiving are sorely needed.[18] In these pages, readers can listen in on the ongoing conversation of a patient and her companion in mortal time and imagine their own journeys toward living at the end.

Notes

1. Barbara Ehrenreich coined the term *Cancerland* in her brilliant essay, "Welcome to Cancerland: A mammogram leads to a cult of pink kitsch" in *Harper's Magazine* (November 2001).

2. McQuellon, R. P., & Cowan, M. A. (2000). Turning toward death together: Conversation in mortal time. *American Journal of Hospice & Palliative Care, 17*(5), 312–318.

3. Eiseley, L. (1971), One night's dying. In *The Night Country*. New York: Charles Scribner and Sons.

4. Vollmann, W. T. (2010, November). A good death: Exit strategies. *Harper's Magazine.*

5. Seng-ts'an. (2014). *Hsin-hsin Ming: Verses on the faith-mind* (R. B. Clarke, Trans.). http://www.mendosa.com/way.html

6. Sulmasy, D. (2006). Spiritual issues in the care of dying patients: ". . . It's okay between me and God." *Journal of the American Medical Association, 296*(11), 1385–1392.

7. Kooser, T. (2000). Sunny and clear. In *Winter morning walks: One hundred postcards to Jim Harrison* (p. 48). Pittsburgh: Carnegie Mellon Press.

8. Classen, C., Butler, L. D., Koopman, C., Miller, E., DiMiceli, S., Giese-Davis, J., Fobair, P., Carlson, R. W., Kraemer, H. C., & Spiegel, D. (2001). Supportive-expressive group therapy and distress in patients with metastatic breast cancer: A randomized clinical intervention trial. *Archives of General Psychiatry, 58*(5), 494–501.

9. Spiegel, D., Bloom, J., Kraemer, H. C., & Gottheil, E. (1989). Effect of psychosocial treatment on patients with metastatic breast cancer. *Lancet, 2*(8668), 888–891.

10. Egan, G. (1994). *The skilled helper* (5th ed.). Belmont, CA: Brooks/Cole Publishing.

11. Lieberman, M. D., Eisenberger, N. I., Crockett, M. J., Tom, S. M., Pfeifer, J. H., & Way, B. M. (2007). Putting feelings into words: Affect labeling disrupts amygdala activity in response to affective stimuli. *Psychological Science, 18*(5), 421–428.

12. Reiss, H. (2018). *The empathy effect: Seven neuroscience-based keys for transforming the way we live, love, work and connect across differences.* Boulder: Sounds True.

13. Chokinov, H. M. (2012). *Dignity therapy: Final words for final days.* Oxford: Oxford University Press.

14. Kagan, N. I., & McQuellon, R. P. (1981). Interpersonal process recall in psychotherapy. In R. J. Corsini (Ed.), *Handbook of innovative psychotherapies* (pp. 443–458). New York: Wiley.

15. McQuellon, R. P. (1982). Interpersonal process recall. In E. K. Marshall & P. D. Kurtz (Eds.), *Interpersonal helping skills* (pp. 161–202). San Francisco: Jossey-Bass.

16. Deborah Laramore, RN, leads the healing touch clinical program at Wake Forest Baptist Health. See https://www.wakehealth.edu/Locations/Clinics/i/Integrative-Medicine-Highland-Oaks.

17. See https://en.wikipedia.org/wiki/Ars_moriendi: "The *Ars moriendi* are two related Latin texts dating from about 1415 and 1450. They offer advice on the protocols and procedures of a good death, explaining how to 'die well' according to Christian precepts of the late Middle Ages."

18. Gawande, A. (2014). *Being mortal: Medicine and what matters in the end.* New York: Henry Holt & Company.

1

February 16, 2005—Seeking Witness

Preparing for death is one of the most profoundly healing acts of a lifetime.

> Levine, S. (1997). *A year to live: How to live this year as if it were your last.* (p. 7). New York: Three Rivers Press.

Main Themes: Radical changes in appearance and life interrupts dying on schedule.

This is the first meeting we recorded and the last in the comprehensive cancer center clinic. The primary theme is readiness for the next step toward death and frustration at its delay.

Nell's physical status is declining rapidly; it is hard for her to get in and out of a car and to walk. Her body is visibly deteriorating, plodding toward death. This is the first time she speaks in depth about the dramatic, frightening changes she sees in her body.

Nonetheless, she jokes about completing her worldly tasks; she has nearly finished her income taxes! She has met with her medical oncologist who confirmed that her death was not imminent. She is disappointed demise is not following her timeline. This theme is common for Nell and occurs throughout our conversations. We have discussed the topic of mortality many times, starting at our initial meeting when she explained her disappointment that breast cancer had not taken her life sooner. She also speaks of comfort from consoling touch and a negative reaction to hospice.

In our previous meeting, I asked Nell how she would feel about recording our conversations. She agreed, and her mood brightened at the idea. We signed the necessary documents. Even though her physical vulnerability is increasing, her confidence in expressing herself is unshaken.

In this dialogue, you learn of Mary, Nell's dear friend, who lives in New York City. She has training in guided imagery, a gentle but powerful method that focuses the imagination in proactive, positive ways. Nell has used it for weeks to manage fear and settle her mind; it is a soothing technique that requires little conversation, except to reflect on the response to the experience, and it connects Nell to her friend. We had used guided imagery in our previous sessions, although Nell prefers to process her feelings in conversation.

Nell is acutely aware of her emaciated body. She longs for a witness to her bodily transformation. We begin with this brave revelation.

Dialogue 1

N: There is something I want to tell you, yet there's nothing you can do about it. I hope someday people caring for cancer patients will make someone available to witness bodily changes from cancer, as part of care for advanced patients, when patients request it.

RM: OK, tell me about it.

N: There is a painful irony here because a time is coming soon when I will have no control over access to my body. There will be other people washing and turning me and changing my diaper, if I don't get out of this world first. (Laughs.) I have played the "washing–changing–turning loved ones" role. The thought of being on the receiving side of it upsets me badly.

RM: You know what that's like, and you recognize that your turn is coming unless you die first?

N: Yes. For the last month, when I get ready to take a shower, I've scrutinized my body in the mirror intensely. I have watched my body change dramatically in such scary ways. I look like a big beetle, a carcass with little stems like arms and legs.

RM: You are transforming, and it's very frightening.

N: My back has no flesh on it, no buns. I am nothing but a huge mass pushing my ribs out. I look like a starvation victim, you know? Bony and bloated. It is so terrifying that I've just about stopped looking.

RM: So hard—a very scary transformation.

N: What I've realized is that I would like a witness—there needs to be a witness—somebody who would say, "Yes, I'm willing to look at that scary thing," if a patient requested it. My body is so frightening to me. I will never ask Al to do it. I don't want to frighten him, too. It's like longing for your lover, for the comfort of someone else sharing your deep fear. And it's not exactly this thing with fear of dying—it's fear of not being heard or seen. I wonder if other patients ever articulate that kind of fear, that kind of loneliness?

RM: Yes, some patients speak of such fear and loneliness. You articulate your feelings clearly. Years ago, I talked with a survivor of the concentration camp at Dachau. She had lost weight and was very thin due to her cancer ordeal. She said, "When I look in the mirror now, I see myself in Dachau." She showed me the tattooed numbers on her forearm. That was her way of grasping the changes caused by her cancer and its treatment. What you have just told me is like that, one of the most powerful statements I have ever heard about the fear evoked by radical appearance changes.

Commentary: *Nell is profoundly vulnerable now, and her revelation registers with me as a message of deep trust. She is terrified by what she sees. She would like a witness to look at her, to share her painful burden. I am a witness to her reflections, with an acute awareness of her bloating body. I am glad she doesn't ask me to look at her. I am aware of the limitations of my role, yet why can't professional boundaries be stretched for a higher purpose? Being Nell's witness in the way she seeks is beyond the role I was trained in as a psychologist, yet, in this moment, she needs a witness, and I have not spoken. Is it enough to listen to her story without viewing her ravaged body? I have encountered this feeling of not doing enough throughout my professional career as a caregiver. I feel it now. Can't I do more?*

N: I never before thought about sight or vision as a form of communication. Looking back to our first conversations about your article, about this place in which we talk, I realized that at least for visual-minded people, maybe it could be a very healing kind of communication. I cannot envision how it would be institutionalized. It would need to be carefully done and respectful to avoid exploitation. I think it could be part of the healing process. I expect that is something that hospice people probably are better at doing?

RM: Yes, hospice workers could be more helpful in witnessing physical changes.

N: Should be. One likes to hope.

Commentary: Nell is referring to an article written by Michael Cowan and me.[1] I had given her a copy early in our meetings. Its central theme is how conversation about mortal time and death can be healing. Shortly after she read it, she sent me a poem she had written about the relief she felt at the thought of my office, this safe haven where she could talk openly about her fears and hopes. We could talk about death. She felt comfort in telling her story from our first meeting. Her positive comment about the therapeutic process reassured me. Recalling the words of my kind, pragmatic father—"Make yourself useful and have compassion for others"—I hope to be useful to Nell.

Nell wrote a poem (Box 1.1) while sitting at Salem Square, a lovely area in the center of Old Salem, the historic site of one of first Moravian settlements in North Carolina, after she had attended Sunday church service.

Box 1.1 Time and Balance

I speak of space—the "space" where we face death, the "space" where we talk together. Maybe every embedded metaphor is like this, taken for granted, elusive head-on. Head-on is grass due for mowing, thick with the shade of mid-autumn trees, shorter in the sunlight. A trick of the eye. Like capturing the moment. The definite edge of the trees formed creeps across the lawn as compactly as my gathered breath ticks within my chest wall.

Capturing the moment, counting the breath, attempting to be in the now. Facing death together. Being in that space.

The solid shadow of a tree just before it loosens every leaf in a glory of fall. Drifting in color. Touching light.

The moment, tremendous moment, when altogether we assent. This is my body, this is my blood. A procession of assents. Each of us a leaf in a glory about to burst in a hail of liberation. Serial steps of life in death.

RM: I'm just thinking about your very profound, thoughtful observation and request about being seen. In the world we live in, even with your good medical team, it would be very unusual. "Look with me and help me understand—tell me about my body." As close as medicine comes to that would be the physician who examines you, and even then, typically, only parts of you are examined.

N: My doctor doesn't examine. He'll palpate, but the story is over as far as examining to find out what's going on. He knows what's going on. And it's not so much me saying, "Look at me and explain what's happened in my body," because I think I've gotten that part. But I'm thinking something more ceremonial and more like grieving. Just grieve with me, so I can move on through this.

RM: The witnessing would be part of your grieving?

N: I haven't thought about that before, but it could be. It would be nice if there were a ceremony.

Commentary: Nell seeks consoling touch and a healing gaze from her professional caregivers, while beginning to understand the limitations of her medical team. She is learning that the conventions of modern medicine usually do not include a conscious effort to make touch emotionally healing. The physician palpates for a functional reason: to diagnose. She rightly observes that he does not examine because he already knows what is happening to her body, yet she seeks a ritual of recognition and compassionate connection during her appointment. She would like at least one person, perhaps her medical oncologist, to join in her story in a different way.[2] Many, if not most, cancer patients have expectations that go unmet partly because they are unrealistic. Nell may not have realized she had such an expectation until she experienced it in the moment. Patients experience disappointment of a different sort when they learn about the inexact science of predicting and managing treatment-related side effects, so highly dependent on the individual and the treatment team's ability to match the symptom to a medication.

RM: What I hear you describing is a ritual letting go of the shell that is your body, a body that is transforming into something that is not recognizable to you.

N: I can hardly look at myself.

RM: The change is hard to see, and yet you are springing from this cocoon. It's starting to wither away. It will not have its standard beauty but a different type. You seek a ritual of witnessing your transformation. Perhaps it could be part of a hospice ritual, should you want?

N: There is only one hospice in this town, isn't there? (Nell grimaces with displeasure.)

RM: Is it a bad one? What is your perspective so far?

N: My experience with it so far. (Frowns, shakes her head.)

RM: What happened?

N: They are the people who ditched me when I was doing marathon vomiting. Because they would not give me Zofran. That's all I needed. It was not in their formulary. They had promised me they could get it when they got me to sign on. This "bait and switch" just pissed me off. They promised me that I could have Zofran even though it was not in their formulary, but the doctor who made that promise . . . was on vacation, and so the doctor who was on just said, "You can wait a week, or you can take the medicine we are prepared to offer you." At this, I realized I was in the hospital in June, where I had landed from dehydration from vomiting. I was right back into vomiting, and this was their answer?

RM: I see where you might say, "Shove it!"

N: Very much so, and what really teed me off was there was no follow-up. I vomited that morning four times before 9 a.m., and [the doctor] said I could not have Zofran. So I called, and a worker—he was like, "Whoops, sorry"—no nurse, no nothing. I didn't know what I was supposed to do—go dehydrate completely or something? Fortunately, I lived through it, and the next week I signed off (laughs) on hospice and wrote a very testy letter that said, "This is not up to your standards, not to mention mine" (laughs).

RM: What kind of response did you get?

N: None from the doctors. Some PR person called and said: "Oh, we are really sorry this happened to you, blah, blah, blah, blah, blah." And they apologized. "We're really sorry, but we're going to do things our way" is the way it came through.

RM: I can see where your reluctance to work with hospice would come in.

N: I am very reluctant to work with hospice. We had a friend who stayed with us. I was her caregiver for years, and she was wasting away from multi-infarct dementia. We brought her home from the nursing home seven months before she died. Hospice started coming. The two things that were troublesome for her were exactly the two things that were troublesome for me in this experience. One was their grip on their formulary, and they were using a mail-order pharmacy in Philadelphia. If the nurse or CNA [certified nursing assistant] or whoever had come out hadn't ordered stuff on time, it never got here because "it's the weekend. We don't pay extra for Fed Ex and blah, blah, blah, blah, blah." You constantly had to urge them to keep the medications current.

Commentary: Nell has been negotiating her own ending at home with spouse Al by her side and close friends available by phone and visits. I am trying to provide additional guidance for her. I place great hope in her physician and our local hospice. A common conundrum in this situation: What is the therapist to do when the patient criticizes a valued colleague or a good resource like hospice? I often walk the line, explaining the limitations of medical care, perhaps seeming to excuse fellow professional caregivers, while validating a patient's observations. I have had many good experiences with hospice and its professionals, and I have great respect for Nell's medical oncologist. Still, I understand how she can become disappointed with care when expectations are not met. I see my role as helping Nell and all my patients to understand the limitations of our providers and our healthcare system. Medicine is a victim of its own success in terms of creating very high expectations for healthcare and, at times, unrealistic expectations for cure. Nell later embraces the fine care she finds with her hospice nurses and aides.

RM: So you have seen a not-so-effective hospice operating?

N: Yes! The other weakness was the quality of the nursing staff who would come out. Naturally, they were the most harried, underpaid human beings in their profession. There was no consistency or continuity. It was just another shell game. An

HMO [health maintenance organization] is basically a great idea, but the execution is wrong. So I have had one substantial experience with hospice and the second one, mercifully short, in another city. It was just rotten quality. I do not want to go back to them. Maybe I want to be very, very quiet. Yet am I not supposed to fear for my weight loss and dying in my bed?

RM: Managing without hospice may be doable. I have a nurse friend who used to work for hospice. She has specialized in helping in these times as you approach the end. She's a special nurse, who knows the body and the spirit. You have encountered the bureaucracy called hospice, perhaps the worst it has to offer. The best it has to offer is trained professionals who know how to help people toward dying in a confident and thoughtful way—the physical, technical piece as well as the spiritual. With regard to the practical, symptom management is key, especially pain medication. I would like to ask my nurse friend about her status and what she might be able to do. Is that OK?

N: Yes, please.

RM: The medical management is one piece. We focus more on the emotional and mental aspects of this process. You are facing death, and you have some idea about dying well. You know that your vision cannot be completed easily without certain people to guide you. Some are coming up short. If they could only give you some peace, reassurance, or a plan—

N: I need a plan, yes! I don't want to drive Al nuts. However, that's not the whole thing. I do not want to be doped up more than I have to and miss the whole transition (laughs).

RM: Absolutely, you are right to avoid being doped up and missing the transition.

N: Yes, I want to be alert and have people help me at the end. It can get to you. The people who write these panegyrics—"Oh, how wonderful hospice is!"—are often, not always, people who don't want to see the suffering, want to think it was painless, want their loved ones doped to the gills. I don't want that. There should be a right to die mindfully! (Laughs.)

RM: You are setting the pace, setting the scene and creating your story, writing your script. You are a good director.

N: My body is telling me what to do, and I am trying to listen to it. The body and my imagery work—both are saying that it is coming, that death is coming at a steady pace, straight for me. (Laughs.) And that's why getting that healthy chunk of the income tax preparation done was helpful. OK, well, that's off the table now, and I have very few things left on the table to complete (chuckles), which is good.

RM: You have made space, and you need space. I have an image of a table with lots of clutter moving off. It is clearer now.

N: Yes. Really, in just the last few weeks, I have found that I can tell myself I am dying, and it has not frightened me. I have just turned some corner. I am not sure what it is, but it is like an endorphin high. It's a resolution. I am no longer afraid of death, and it's not that I talked myself into it. I feel as if it is something that my body is ready to face—my body, not my mind.

RM: Your body is the shell. You are living toward death mindfully. Your goal—to be at home in bed with Al by your side and others with you as you make the transition—is reasonable.

N: I hope so, but I know there are no guarantees.

RM: Yes, there may be another scene, too, if you should need more medical care and pain management. This is where the technical, symptom management piece is key because medical care on site can be important. Just to give you this notion—you may have yourself set up, ready to go, and all of a sudden, you get intractable pain, and you are shipped to the hospital. That is possible. Keep in mind these various pathways.

N: If they ship me to the "Hospice Inn," that, I think, would be a different kind of impression.

RM: Would you like that?

N: I think it would be OK, if necessary. But I wouldn't want to go to hospice just because I could not get my book off the shelf or something like that. (Laughs.) It would be a little harder to control creature comforts like that at hospice, but heck, I really don't think it's all that important.

RM: You are doing well seeking your comfort zone. It is a good balance between seeking and letting things be.

N: That's welcome.

RM: You are seeking what I hope for you or myself and my loved ones—a home to launch from. The only thing that could avert that might be the necessity for more intensive pain management. The next best spot might be inpatient hospice with appropriate care. You're listening to your body. You do not seem to be hastening or avoiding. Both your humor and sadness are alive. You are not afraid of your grief. What do you think?

N: Yes, and what I am surprised by is how much of this knowledge comes nonverbally. That's what it's starting to do to me. The body is contributing to the body/mind play here. I brought this little Post-it Note tablet. Mary and I still talk at great length, but I do not keep a journal anymore. I just do not have the energy. But I grabbed a Post-it and wrote this down on the 8th of February. (Chuckles.) This is almost a review, a sort of recapitulation. One, this cancer is not just an illness. It is a process, and I find that a very liberating thought. Cancer is a bodily process that went all screwed up, cells multiplying out of control. (Chuckles.) Two, the tumor is an agent; it is not the enemy. That's a good thing. If something is taking up half of your food supply and all of your body (chuckles), and you are living it, it's important to identify your relationship with it. (Hearty laugh.) And three, I am not responsible for the frustration of this process! (Laughs.)

RM: Beautiful!

Commentary: Nell summarizes her understanding of cancer with three wise observations. This wisdom will help to guide her in the weeks to come. Seeing cancer as a process—a series of experiences and actions leading to a particular end—allows her to proceed with purpose. Recognizing the tumor as an agent allows her to avoid the war metaphor, which is anathema to Nell. She does not embrace the notion that cancer is an enemy to be battled, which is the default position our culture offers to people facing serious illness.[3] Finally, recognizing the inherent frustration in the process of managing her cancer allows her to anticipate what is to come.

N: I think these observations of cancer fit with my experience. (Laughs.) I thought number three was just absolutely heaven because I get very frustrated. I see my friends and loved ones being frustrated, and then I feel responsible. "Oh dear, I don't want to upset so-and-so," or "Oh dear, I'm getting boring."

RM: Yes, it is a hard habit to let go of—feeling responsible for loved ones' feelings.

N: Mary is a jewel. She has helped me with these insights.

RM: Yes, she is a real jewel. Now, we have work to do. I am going to make a call to my nurse colleague and ask her about meeting with you. Regarding our meetings, we should have Plan A and B. Plan A—we meet up in a week here in the cancer center. Plan B—I will come to your home, if you decide you're not getting around well enough to come in.

N: Thank you.

Final Commentary: Nell is not alone in calling for recognition of her physical metamorphosis, for a witness. Some courageous women have called others to witness their mutilating surgeries in graphic photos. In "The Warrior" poster, breast cancer patient Deena Metzger poses exuberantly, revealing her tree branch tattoo over her mastectomy scar. The poster is a collaboration among Metzger, photographer Hella Hammid, and graphic designer Sheila de Bretteville.[4] Matuschka, a renowned fashion model and activist, was one of the first women to display her mastectomy scar, on the cover of the New York Times

Magazine.[5] *Both Metzger and Matuschka were brave pioneers helping to raise consciousness/awareness of breast cancer.*

Professor Mary DeShazer synthesized a large portion of women's cancer literature in her scholarly work Fractured Borders.[6] *DeShazer reflects on ways in which women's ill bodies have been textually represented: medicalized bodies, leaking bodies, amputated bodies, prosthetic bodies, and finally surviving bodies. Nell's body was changing dramatically. While it does not fit easily into any one of these categories, she very eloquently described how her bloating, changing body frightened her. It was ravaged and traumatized by the relentless growth of metastatic breast cancer. At one point here, she made a distinction between body and mind; she felt her body was ready to die, but her mind was not, a point we will come back to in future conversations.*

Nell is seeking the "click of contact" so well described by Anatole Broyard in his essay "The Patient Examines the Doctor."[7] The click comes when eye contact signals a powerful moment of understanding and empathic human connection, when the doctor is more than a role and the patient more than a number on a list.

I wonder if I could have done more for Nell, yet I find some comfort in recalling these words from the autobiography of Zora Neale Hurston, referenced by poet Maya Angelou: "There is no greater agony than bearing an untold story inside of you."[8] I can hear and tell Nell's story. Is it enough to listen to her speak about her ravaged body? Reading the transcripts allows me to see how many possible conversational pathways could have been followed, paths that I chose not to take or overlooked entirely. In our next conversation, Nell reveals the effects of talking about yearning for a witness.

Notes

1. McQuellon, R. P., & Cowan, M. A. (2000). Turning toward death together: Conversation in mortal time. *American Journal of Hospice & Palliative Care, 17*(5), 312–318.

2. Novelist Tobias Wolff provides an excellent concept of story: "We live by stories. It's the principle by which we organize our experience and thus derive our sense of who we are. We're in an unceasing flow of time and events and people, and to make sense of what goes past, we put a beginning and an end to a certain thing, and we leave things out and we heighten other things, and in that way we break the unbroken flow into stories, because that's the only way we can give it significance." Quoted in Keillor, G. (2020, June 19). *Writer's Almanac.* http://www.garrisonkeillor.com/radio/twa-the-writers-almanac-for-june-19-2020/

3. Kuner, S., Orsborn, C., Quigley, L., & Stroup, K. (1999). *Speak the language of healing: Living with breast cancer without going to war (New approach to breast cancer).* Newburyport, MA: Red Wheel; and Sulik, G. (2011). *Pink ribbon blues: How breast cancer culture undermines women's health.* New York: Oxford University Press. Nell, like many patients, did not find the war metaphor useful. She was not doing battle but was rather engaged in a relationship with her breast cancer.

4. Jewish Women's Archive. (n.d.). Deena Metzger as the warrior poster. https://jwa.org/media/warrior-poster

5. Matuschka. (1988, August). "You can't look away anymore." *New York Times Magazine.* Quoted in Ferraro, S. (1993, August 15). The anguished politics of breast cancer. *New York Times Magazine.* https://www.nytimes.com/1993/08/15/magazine/the-anguished-politics-of-breast-cancer.html

6. DeShazer, M. K. (2005). *Fractured borders: Reading women's cancer literature.* Ann Arbor: University of Michigan Press.

7. Broyard, A. (1992). The patient examines the doctor. In *Intoxicated by my illness and other writings on life and death.* New York: Clarkson Potter.

8. Hurston, Z. N. (1942). *Dust tracks on a road: An autobiography.* New York: Harper Collins.

2

March 23, 2005—Getting Finished

Stories are medicine . . . They have such power; they do not
require that we do, be, act anything—we need only listen.

Estes, C. P. (1992). *Women who run with the
wolves: Myths and stories of the wild woman
archetype* (p. 15). New York: Ballantine Books.

Main Themes: Disappointment at her too-slow movement toward
death and spiritual concerns.

Since our last meeting nearly a month ago, Nell had increased
contact with home hospice care, a big step taken with the encouragement of her medical team. I want to help her to understand what
she can realistically expect from hospice and her medical team,
especially with regard to the practical aspects of care, including
symptom management and self-advocacy.

Tumor growth has made outings increasingly difficult for her.
Previously, we made plans to meet in her home should her mobility
be further impaired. I have made home visits before when patients
became incapacitated.

Most of Nell's interactions with healthcare providers and other
caregivers were helpful, but some were troubling. Her physician
had disappointed her by saying that death was not yet on the near
horizon, even though she was retaining fluid. At our first meeting
months ago, her primary complaint was that death was not moving
quickly enough to suit her, an uncommon perspective.

In this dialogue, Nell muses about spiritual concerns. She finds her journey toward death surprising and worries that the power of her life force may be prolonging her earth time. Even though irritability affects her relationships, her humor remains alive. She begins our conversation with disappointment at the timeline of her death.

Dialogue 2

N: I was saying last time we met that having done all this death-and-dying work, we have it all kind of figured out and gotten positioned, and the bed is right, the room is right, and I've done all my jobs—the income tax is done—I've labeled the clothes in the closet, who they should go to. Anyway, I want to get finished. It's like hanging around after the last act, but the last act has not finished!

RM: Yes, not quite there. It's a long act.

N: My deflation with Dr. T this morning was learning that I do not have what is truly needed to die. I do have these big pockets of edema in my legs. The hospice nurse is nice, and she explained that as your organs shut down, they fail to process fluid, and the fluids back up and occupy these positions. It's known as dependent edema. I told her my feelings about that—that it was good. We are making progress on our last task, which is to die, right? That is the last task.

RM: Yes, you are making good progress. Yet, you said "deflation" with Dr. T?

N: I was looking forward to Dr. T saying, yes, that's right, that's what we're doing! Instead, he just said, "Well, that's a generalization. In your case, it's the liver." He was not directly contradicting what the hospice nurse said, but it was taking the punch out of it because he was giving it a very, very gradual and a very indefinite timeline. This could go on for a long time. I was disappointed. I wanted him to say, "Yay team! You're approaching the finish line here. You're just about done, and this is how you can tell—you've already just poofed up with un-processed fluids, and you will quietly sleep away."

RM: So somehow the journey, the path that you are imagining, it's not turning out the way you anticipated?

N: Yes! Here's my concern. You remember last summer we struggled with this because the "six month-ers" were wrong, and here was Nell still tooling along. That's kind of fun and interesting for a while, but it's getting in my way. My question is this: Am I keeping myself alive, perversely, by being capable of getting interested in things all the time? I'm always capable of reading a book by a new author that I like a lot, going to the computer and getting everything else she wrote from Barnes & Noble, and reading the rest of it or something like that. There is always more there to be excited about in the world, always. Am I defeating my own purpose now by continuing to be so excitable? I suppose it is part of my karma because that's just who I am. I have to stay with who I am even if it disappoints me by keeping me where I do not much want to be, which is alive with my unfinished assignment!

Commentary: At our very first meeting, Nell startled me by saying she was disappointed because the six-month expiration date her physician predicted had come and gone, and she was still very much alive. She had hoped for a death that would allow her to avoid seeing her husband deteriorate due to Alzheimer's. Now, Nell is disappointed once again since she has completed the psycholog-ical preparatory work for launching to the next world—she is ready to let go— and, to her surprise, her physician says she is not in im-minent danger, even though her physical appearance has changed radically, including a bulging tumor in her liver. Nell would like her doctor to predict her lifespan, to tell her that she should not buy green bananas because she will not live long enough to see them ripen. She is experiencing the inherent tension in holding on to the things she loves and letting go of life.[1] *Must we let go of our worldly interests in order to die peacefully? I do not know what to say to Nell, and nod in agreement.*

RM: It is your style to be engaged. What I hear you saying is your life is getting in the way of your dying.

N: Perfect! Exactly. My life is getting in the way of my death.

RM: And it is a good life, as I see it.

N: It's a fine life, really. I am sorry to say that (laughs). I guess that it just means that we are infinitely adaptable. I am totally at home in bed, on the phone, reading, television, DVDs. It's all a removed kind of life, but it is still my life. Those hours when I'm awake, I cannot do intellectual work. I cannot work on issues like I did with my dissertation. In a stronger state, I would go develop ideas or something like that. I cannot do that kind of thinking. However, I certainly can read a book, visit with a friend, and talk about the book and so forth.

RM: You are very much alive and yet changing.

N: Yes, I'm turning into a cranky person, which I don't like. I suppose my emotional nerves, like my bodily nerves, do not have any sheathing or protection anymore. I notice it here very, very much. There are spots in this floor and downstairs where the noise level is incredibly high, and I just have to shut down completely until I get out of there, or I'm like tense and on edge, on my last nerve. It feels like that with people, too. When the energy runs out, it's just out. I can just barely be polite because the energy's all gone. I don't have a secure grip on those devices that we count on to buffer out little social irritations. I have to be really, really careful not to be snappish with people I love for no other reason than that I am just worn out.

RM: And what if you were snappish?

N: Well, then I'd have to crawl and apologize in Al's case because I know that things hurt him disproportionately now. It's not easy for him to just blow it off if I'm snappish with him. That would be very hard, so I have to really struggle with myself not to do that to him.

Commentary: Nell's usual pattern of interpersonal communication is changing along with her moods, which she describes as "cranky" and "snappish." She struggles with the yo-yo process of how to be both together with and apart from her caregivers, especially Al. She does not want to offend or hurt him. What she longs for now is a companion who will sit, quietly present, and let her be, yet Al needs her acknowledgment.

The needs of patients and caregivers often diverge during cancer care and can be a source of tension that calls for honest, open interpersonal communication. Her observation recalls the difficulty in adhering to the principle she named in Chapter 1: "I am not responsible for the feelings of others." However, she feels responsible for Al's feelings, a longtime pattern in their relationship. A simple strategy to meet her needs while being sensitive to Al's may be all that is required. I suggest a way to let him know when she needs to be alone.

In the following exchange, we shift to problem-solving along with empathic listening. The two are not mutually exclusive; one can facilitate the other. Problem-solving without empathy can be rejected as a command delivered without mutual, accurate understanding of the situation.

RM: You do not want to push him away, yet that's part of the irritability—whether or not you're living or dying, irritability can push people away. You are doing the work of leaving the world. You have to shove off.

N: That is a perfect paradox. I have to stop being interested in so many people. It is part of leaving the world, and yet I don't want to leave the world grouchy. You don't want to hurt the people who have been so loving and kind to you, like unbelievable Anna.[2] She's awesome. And she brought me reading material. She's just thinking ahead all the time how to make things better for me.

RM: Anna is helpful and nonetheless you are irritable. Tell me about your crankiness.

N: To be fair, I just want to be alone. I feel like there is a process going on. I guess my dying process is the work, in a sense, because I'm doing work now. And it runs parallel to whatever is going on in the moment. Even talking with you, it's still going on, like a factory humming in the background. At the end of the day, when there have been two or three long phone calls and two or three visits, that's when I really want to be alone. But some of the time, it's just a feeling of needing to be closed and quiet. I can be very ambivalent because, on the one hand, I often want the comfort of someone nearby. Anna's perfect because Anna can be nearby and sit and read. She can be nearby and not be intrusive. When Al is nearby, he sits and doesn't bring something to read, and he sits, and I have a feeling as though he is waiting for me to be interested. Then I close my eyes and pretend that I'm falling asleep so that he will go away. (Laughs.) Because I just don't feel responsible to entertain. I'm muddling. I feel as if I'm rambling about little muddles that I'm in all the time, but that is the process.

Commentary: These remarks are a concrete example of how Nell is letting go of the people she loves. Later in our dialogues, she decides to abandon emailing, letting go of another way she has been engaged in the world of interpersonal relationships.

RM: It doesn't sound like rambling. I hear you describing interactions that are the sandpaper of living, grating on you periodically. You have one caregiver who knows how to be with you. This is either a skill Al never had, or it's something he is unable to do now. He may be expecting something from your direction, and that's not what you have to give him right now. You need time for peaceful restfulness. Does Al know how you feel?

N: If he has a clue, then he's never shown a sign of it.

RM: I wonder if it's as simple as letting it be or saying, "Al, I want to take a rest now. I'll call you in a bit." Is it that simple, or is there something else? This may seem like a muddle, but it's important. You had three calls and three visits—that's a lot.

N: A lot of focusing on people.

RM: It takes energy to focus on others, and today you want to withdraw. You are going within. Occasionally people interrupt your flow by expecting something from you, and that's what doesn't feel right.

N: That's right, it doesn't feel right. It's not that I'm sophisticated about my feelings at all. It's as simple as it doesn't feel right. I wish I knew. I have a feeling that we all know forward as much as we know backward. If we could somehow hear the processes of our body-mind, we would know everything that we need to know about the future. I get a sense of having an assignment. The task now is finishing the task of living! My sense is that I'm just about there. It's why I got really deflated when Dr. T didn't say, "Good girl! You're getting there! One more good push and you should make it!" (Laughs.)

Commentary: When Nell said, "We all know forward as much as we know backward," I wondered what she meant. Was she saying if only she could access the body's wisdom, she would know her path toward death? I was thinking, "Does she know how wise she is now? If she could only hear her inner wisdom, understand the processes of her own body-mind, perhaps she would know everything she needs to know about her hoped-for future. This goal is laudable but difficult, perhaps impossible, to achieve.

RM: Well, that's it, you're in labor. And you're thinking the doctor, instead of sitting around, should give you something to speed up delivery. He disappointed you with his explanation of your edema and saying that it's your liver that is going to cause the difficulties, not edema.

N: He was saying the edema has two processes, one due to in-activity and the other, the failure of the liver. He didn't deny that the liver is failing, but he said this is the same process. He went on to say this is the process we've have been looking at all along, and it's not changed substantially. And he said, "You know I've told you, it's nothing dramatic; it's something just very gradual and undramatic." I just do not want to go on and on in these little increments each time.

RM: When you say go on and on, what do you mean?

N: That I'll just keep going at the level I'm going at, the level of function that I'm at right now. I feel as if I just about have the courage up to die, and I think, "I've started." I have started to think about actually dying, not only all that we've been doing approaching this leap, but the leap out of this world itself—letting my mind get exposed to letting that happen. I can't dwell on it because when I do, an involuntary fear ripples through me. That was a big step for me in imagination, and I guess I cannot teeter there all the time.

Commentary: When Nell speaks of an "involuntary fear ripple," I recognize the onset of a similar sensation in myself. As a result of our conversations, I have been thinking more about death, sometimes with an electric surge of apprehension. Being close to Nell triggers my own anxiety. It invariably appears when she directly contemplates her own death, a place of inherent tension. While she struggles with it, I try to understand and reflect on her current state without suggesting that there is a clear path toward dying, especially at home. Practical, medical, interpersonal, and psychological factors must be managed. I wonder if Nell will be able to pull it off, but I keep my questions to myself, preferring to reflect her feelings back to her.

RM: There is a kind of inherent tension, fear, in that place, and you cannot perch there indefinitely. You can think of your life unfolding at the end in hours to days, days to weeks, or perhaps weeks to months. You are transitioning, eyes open, looking around, and understanding. In some ways, you've outpaced your death. You are psychologically, emotionally, spiritually prepared. It seems you have done the work.

N: It seems?

RM: Yes, it seems to me that way. The only reason I say "seems" is that maybe your body, mind, spirit has something to do yet. It's not quite finished. That's a possibility. But that doesn't seem to be the case to me because you've already done the great forgiveness in your life with your father and Al. I just offer this as a way of understanding the inexplicable. What do you think?

Commentary: The "great forgiveness" is a topic we discussed periodically over the months of therapy. It refers to forgiving two important people in Nell's life: her father for the mistreatment she felt and Al for his lack of emotional presence over the years. This theme was common in our earlier sessions but eased over the months as she began to appreciate fully what Al could bring to their marriage.

When I said "it seems" in reference to preparing for death, Nell was perplexed. I think she felt I was saying perhaps she was not ready, it only seemed so. I said she might have some business to complete and, in doing so, confronted my own doubts about comments/statements professionals and relatives make when an unconscious person lingers at the doorstep of death: "She's waiting for her son to come before she lets go," or "you need to tell her it's OK to go." Could the body hold on to life so tenaciously, without regard for the psychological disposition of the patient? Nell regularly affirms that she is ready to die, yet death remains on the horizon. While her worldly tasks are nearly completed, her body is functioning well given its tumor burden. What is keeping her here?

N: That's helpful. Because it maintains that intimacy with myself. You were asking me what I sense. My sense is soon. My sense is that I'm nearly there. I hope the body's on board for this. You know?

RM: What do you mean, hoping the body's on board?

N: Well, I hope I'm not just deluding myself in my multiple selves as we talk to each other. The body-mind connection. I hope that my material body remembers that it's part of the act.

RM: It doesn't just continue on—in other words, confound the predictions once again. A six-month prediction, and then on and on you go?

N: Yes, yes!

RM: I don't think we are in for that—the kind of confounding that occurred at your initial diagnosis and following.

N: Good.

RM: No, absolutely not. I suppose there is a miracle that could happen, but I think your body is moving toward the great leap.

N: My body is a mess—it really is. It is things like the edema, which is very, very uncomfortable. I have to be driven everywhere. It's just little bits of blood—my nose bleeds and my bottom bleeds. I vomited yesterday, and there was blood in my vomit. It's hard—it's just—it's dying—my body is dying.

RM: Your body is dying, Nell. You are feeling and seeing it more and more.

N: Yes. My sister sent me a CD of photos the family had taken in May when they came to load up the furniture. I thought I was sick in May, but I looked like a fashion model then. I just looked fashionably thin in the photos compared to now. I look like a wraith.

RM: You are much thinner for sure. I know your drastic change in physical appearance has called forth from you the question of being seen and being looked at, of looking at yourself. Your wish for a witness. How is that now?

N: Talking with you about it seemed to accomplish "needing to be seen," the part that I thought was unfinished. Another thing that is very helpful is that the hospice nurses look at me. We look together at things very un-self-consciously and without drama. That is helpful. It's better than I am used to. It is a very subtle difference from the hospital experience, where they only look at what you point out to them. Now, I have gotten more emaciated this last week and a half, and I hoped talks about it with the nurses would come. Just to be fair, Dr. T—he isn't looking at me critically. Yet looking at all of me is not how he sees his job now. So maybe he didn't get that part?

RM: Yes, maybe.

Commentary: *Nell reflects on how hospice personnel can look at her emaciated body, something she had longed for from her medical team, as we discussed at our last meeting. Her wish to be seen by her caregivers no longer troubles her.*

When she spoke of how her body was deteriorating, I thought of a line from Shakespeare's play Cymbeline: *"Golden lads and girls all must as chimney sweepers come to dust" (Act 4, Scene 2, l. 258). Such a reflection might seem morbid, so I keep it to myself. Many thoughts and responses spring to mind in therapy sessions. My task is to offer helpful comments informed by professional training and experience and tact while remaining spontaneous. To hear her say that talking about her troubling feelings helped was a validation of the therapeutic process.*

N: I certainly hope that I'm dying faster than he thinks I am as of this last visit with him. (Laughs.) Of course, the previous visit he seemed to think I was dying faster than I thought!

RM: That's right. The last time we talked, it was just after you heard the "You need to accept hospice care" message.

N: Right. Well, we are reading tea leaves here. Who knows?—it just could be he didn't get his morning snack, or he did, or something else was influencing his judgment about my ending. (Laughs.)

Commentary: One of Nell's best coping methods is her sense of humor. She laughs when she says, "I certainly hope that I am dying faster than my doctor thinks I am!" Ironically and humorously, she suggests that her beloved physician's moods or even snacks might affect his recommendations regarding hospice! Her humor and appreciation for irony help me to remain hopeful in the midst of our serious conversation. It can be sad. It is sad, not depressing, yet it exacts a toll on the listener.

RM: Your sense of humor is very much alive. I believe it will be intact forever.

N: (Laughs.) Well, I hope so.

RM: Just back to the point of being seen—it sounds like the team of hospice nurses is good. I know my colleague-friend with hospice experience has been with you, too. Are they both meeting your standards?

N: The LPN is better than the RN on this team in terms of executing. I think the RN turned me over to the LPN. I understand how to bang the cage when I need food or water. For example, I was very anxious, I couldn't relax about this business of the pain patch until there was a first delivery. So last Friday, I told the RN I just had two patches left to last 72 hours. It's time to order the patch because I don't want to be without it. "Oh, well," she said, "it'll wait until Monday." Monday is not a day to plan to do something because it's always the busiest day. I called her voicemail on Monday to remind her to order the patch and asked her to call me back. Never heard from her. Tuesday, I called and let the triage nurse have the question, "Would you please be sure to get the patch here because now I'm on my last patch that will last 72 hours?" Of course, the triage nurse was in a meeting.

RM: Our triage nurse or the hospice nurse?

N: Hospice nurse. In other words, instead of asking for her voicemail, I said I needed a prescription refill. The receptionist put me through to the triage nurse's voicemail. I said I'm on my last patch, have to have it, please let me know. Well, the triage nurse calls back and says the nurse is coming out to see you. She will take care of your issue. I said, "My what?" because I was half-asleep. Also, I was nervous because of the lack of specificity of "your issue." She said, "Oh, about your prescription refill." Then the nurse called to say that this was the LPN, that she was coming, so I said, "Oh, good, then you can bring my prescription." She said, "Oh, no—the pharmacist delivers the prescription separately." Right about now, I'm thinking all those old jokes (laughs)—how many doctors does it take to refill a prescription?

RM: (Laughs) OK.

 N: But some of my best friends are doctors, OK? (Laughs.) But the LPN came to visit. I said, "Oh, do you have my prescription?" She said, "No, but I remembered that it was important to you, so I went upstairs to the pharmacy, and they hadn't filled it yet. They said that they would get it to you by the end of the day; it would be after work because they were backed up." Now we are going from Friday to Tuesday. It altered my day entirely. Meds should not be an issue. Now, if I hadn't been physically able to take that initiative, I would have been without the patch. That kind of micro-management from the patient shouldn't be in the equation. It's not right.

RM: Yes, I agree. Does the nurse that I recommended know about this?

 N: No, I don't think so. I don't think I told her.

RM: Does the hospice nurse know about it?

 N: I haven't seen the hospice nurse since then. It was the LPN in the afternoon. I sat her down and said, "Look, it shouldn't be like this. I can't afford the anxiety, and you certainly don't need to have an emergency because something routine isn't being treated. How do we manage this? I need your help." We agreed that once a week, she would go over the meds with me for the next week. Well, you know, that's supposed to be what she does anyway, right? We came up with this brilliant idea that is standard of care! (Laughs.)

RM: You are training a lot of people, aren't you?

N: I thought what I would do is ask my private-duty nurse if she would do exactly the same thing once a week and have my back on that. I do not want to always manage my medications because I can't take that much aggravation.

RM: You are holding up your part. Sometimes, other people aren't. All they have to do is listen to you. Thank goodness you speak clearly, and they are kind.

N: They are nice and kind and especially the LPN. They both have nice personalities, but the LPN will take time and talk with you. The RN—you really do have the feeling that she has her 15 minutes and a big patient list.

RM: You have well-tuned antennae for nonverbal cues like "I've got to get out of here. You're bothering me with all your questions." You have a talent for reading nuanced communication. A colleague of mine called it a "crap detector." You have an excellent crap detector, and you use it to assure good care.

N: (Laughs.) I hope so. I think Dr. T partly misinterpreted my question this morning, and I don't know a better way to have put it. I think—because there was a point where he said his mission was to keep me comfortable, but that he did not want any part of hastening death. I tried to be very clear that's not what I was asking for. Maybe I wasn't clear enough, or maybe it's just a very sensitive topic?

RM: It certainly could be, with all the commotion in the news, with the Schiavo decision.[3]

N: Her wishes are demonstratively well known. The authority of her husband. It's been the delusion of the parents.

Commentary: *At no time did Nell ever consider physician-assisted suicide, which she makes clear in our next dialogue.*

RM: It's a reflection of how we do not easily let go. You are doing the work of letting go, not without irritations, not without disappointments. The major forgiveness, the life-review pieces, are coming into place. You may be on the launching pad before you want to be there. Maybe there are some things to review, look at, or simply live with along the way these days?

N: That's probably true. I was thinking—I just finished reading a collection of short stories by Alice Munro, whom I've never read before.[4] She's Canadian. I've spent a lot of time in Ontario—she knows the country. It is largely a very unsupportive landscape, and it isn't generous to life. It was scraped clean by the glacier. You cannot make an easy living there. And the climate is very hard. Her characters are correspondingly spare emotionally, culturally. She's not scary like Margaret Atwood, another great Canadian woman writer. What struck me, paradoxically, about finishing that collection was how affirming it was to me, how life-affirming reading her stories was. I think it was partly that there was life in this very unsupportive environment. There was something worth describing and paying attention to. Her artistry is wonderful.

RM: The work of Alice Munro has made a big impact on you.

N: Oh, she's out there—her new book, which has gotten a lot of attention, is the one I read. It's just in connection with reading that book last week, realizing that the work of being alive is never stopped. But that's back to my present quandary (laughs), which is: I am going to be dying!

Commentary: *Nell's active mind is always looking for connections. In this case, she sees in the work of Alice Munro how someone can remain alive even in the most barren environment. I wonder if she feels she is somehow clinging to life even as her body becomes barren and nearly uninhabitable?*

RM: I have often asked myself, "What would I do?" Would I simply stop eating? But then the hunger pangs and thirst might speak otherwise. People around me might speak otherwise. It might not be very kind to be leaving on my own. What is one to do? Wait? You have done more than wait, living these weeks. From what you have said to me and your physical changes, your spirit is ready. You are ready. You are finishing, teaching, teaching me a great deal. You will leave your voice with me.

N: Yes, thank you.

Final Commentary: *The dialogue regarding pain medication calls to mind a question that has been with me over the course of my career: Why is strong self-advocacy often needed to receive good care? In Nell's case, she is advocating for getting pain medications on time. Should that be necessary? I'm annoyed, yet I understand how delays can occur in the most efficient of systems. It was no time for me to offer a lame explanation for the problems of working through the bureaucracy. Nell is adjusting to the hospice bureaucracy and to the kind nurses who care for her. She is ambivalent about the institution yet very pleased with the interpersonal contact with the nurses who come to her home.*

The final exchanges in this night's conversation make me wonder about my own ending, a topic that is constantly with me while working so closely with Nell. While she sees me as her guide, I see her as my conversation partner, teaching me how to engineer a good death, should I be so fortunate. To this end, our conversations are both enlightening and possibly prophetic.

In our next conversation, Nell reveals her delight in finally feeling at home in the world, pleasantly surprised at her emerging narrative in mortal time.

Notes

1. Gawande, A. (2014). *Being mortal: Medicine and what matters in the end.* New York: Henry Holt.
2. Anna is a close friend and caregiver who provides bedside companionship for several hours two or three times a week.

3. From 1990 to 2005, a right-to-die legal case embroiled the United States. Theresa Marie Schiavo was in an irreversible vegetative state. Her husband and legal guardian argued that she would not have wanted prolonged artificial life support without the prospect of recovery and elected to remove her feeding tube. Schiavo's parents disputed her husband's assertions and challenged her medical diagnosis, arguing in favor of continuing artificial nutrition and hydration. The highly publicized and prolonged series of legal challenges presented by her parents, which ultimately involved state and federal politicians up to the level of President George W. Bush, caused a seven-year delay before Schiavo's feeding tube was removed.

4. Munro, A. (2004). *Runaway*. New York: Vintage.

3

April 5, 2005—Living in Mortal Time

The cost of a thing is the amount of what I will call life which is required to be exchanged for it, immediately or in the long run.

Thoreau, H. D. (1960) *Walden* (p. 25–26)
New York: The New American Library of
World Literature, Signet Classics.

Main Theme: Exploring the meaning of mortal time.

In this dialogue, Nell describes her experience of extended mortal time. This unique, unexpected transition stage allows her to review and reflect on her relationships over her lifetime. Her sense of humor is active even as she recounts experiences of physical discomfort and contemplates death. She finds comfort in the rituals of the church and has referred to herself as "a fitfully practicing Catholic." She appreciates the sacrament of the Anointing of the Sick, while at the same time she has questions about the institutional church and the many problems stemming from patriarchy.

The themes of practical problems (managing a deteriorating body) and soaring toward transcendence (contemplating pure love as the reward on "the other side") coexist. Nell is making peace with her time on earth; the "when" of her death is no longer so pressing for her. Lying passively in wait is a thankless, harrowing, exhausting chore that can lead to great angst. In contrast, Nell is very much alive and actively engaged in her life as it comes to an end. Her spiritual musings encompass the surprises on her journey, including finally feeling at home in the world, and a profound insight about what awaits on the other side.

Dialogue 3

N: I reread your paper today because you were coming. I'm impressed by how important it is, what you are trying to deal with.[1] I said this to you after I read it the first few times: One of the things that intrigues me about this mortal time with cancer is how long it is. You're not rushing to the bedside of someone who has only three days to live. There is essentially a whole evolution that can have an integrity of its own in the time from diagnosis to death. That's an additional narrative.

RM: Thank you for your kind words. Sounds like you are now exploring your new mortal time zone.

N: Yes. There's the narrative of the life, and there's the narrative of the transition in my life. Potentially, I could turn my face to the wall like Hezekiah or someone and say, "Life is over." On the other hand, you could do what we have been doing—trying to explore this space to see what can be done there in terms of growing.

RM: This is new space and has both possibility for growth and dangers to be avoided, to turn away from. You are doing a great job of exploring, growing, and teaching.

N: Well, I hope that my oncologist did not think I was trying to hasten my death when we talked last time. In a sense, I am trying to envision this space/time that is being given to me.

Commentary: Nell was disappointed with her medical oncologist when he did not confirm that the end was imminent. He misinterpreted her intentions, thinking she might want him to assist her in hastening death, yet she did not correct him. Patients who can contradict their physicians in a direct encounter are rare; even articulate patients can fall mute in the examination room. Nell might have been the exception, given her high health literacy. She remained silent even though she never contemplated physician-assisted suicide. Physician-assisted suicide is legal in nine states; nevertheless, it remains controversial, and many healthcare providers are uncomfortable discussing it.

RM: You are a very unusual patient for Dr. T. I don't know how many patients he has known in his career who faced into their own death like you.

N: I cannot imagine *not* wanting to do that. It's a one-time experience. (Laughs.) I have to tell you—I've had three strong experiences lately. They seem to form a chain or build on one another in this process of growing. The first one, I have told you about. It was just a simple, one-day realization that I feel at home in the world. That is stunning to me. I have never felt at home really, yet, after all these decades of trying to find my place in the world, I just suddenly realized that I now know. I do not feel like a stranger in the world or alien. I feel at home.

Commentary: A sense of finally being at home in the world, even as her last act is unfolding, is a profound experience. This feeling has been gradually dawning over the course of our conversations. Nell has made peace with her painful family history and previously unfulfilled hopes for her marriage. She has begun to connect with Al on a deeper level.[2] Following her diagnosis, when she felt an increased need for closeness in her primary relationship, she felt its absence even more acutely. This theme can emerge even in relationships where emotional intimacy has been the norm over the years. The experience of life-threatening illness can be isolating. Being sick, removed from work life and customary roles (e.g., tennis partner, book club member, church member/ attendee), is lonely. Nell has mastered her feeling of alienation in the midst of loss and isolation. She is arriving home. The theme of home recurs throughout our conversations as Nell's body and needs change.

RM: Yes, feeling at home must be a relief.

N: Well, yes, it is. The second realization came about more recently. Suddenly, the mental ticker tape that keeps a chronology going in my mind all the time—stopped. The burden of time—that marginal tally in my head that says, "I'm not dead yet" (laughs) and "Oh, when am I going to get dead? I'm tired of waiting" or "I'm tired of not knowing," mostly not knowing, that stuff which is somehow background noise—suddenly, there was a breakthrough like you get when you finally master a tennis stroke. After months of practice, a particular stroke suddenly comes naturally. You are not breaking down into parts, and you are not struggling with your grip and the rotation of the racket or whatever. You just hit the ball. You hit it right, and it feels right. I tumbled into ease with being mortal. I said to myself, "OK, so I don't know. OK, so it's going to happen when I don't know to brace for it." Just being comfortable with that, not being angry, resentful, or tearful or even particularly curious. The anxiety just fell away. I am just falling into comfortability with being mortal.

Commentary: *Nell is no longer plagued by the intrusive question, "When will I die?" Hearing her calm, open acceptance of death is gratifying. Having addressed the important questions at the end, she is ready.*[3] *She is remarkably resilient in the shadow of her own ending. I wonder if she is avoiding her feelings of loss and sadness since she is strongly attached to the wonders of this world. I admire her and am thankful for her courage. I hope I can approach death like Nell should I have the challenge and gift of lengthy mortal time. I have always assumed I would die suddenly of a massive heart attack like my father, who died at age 46. I am now marching toward death slowly, vicariously, with Nell.*

RM: That's unusual for you, not to be curious.

N: Yes! (Laughs.) I want to tell you about the third realization—a really wonderful one. It happened this morning. I was tired last night and still adjusting to the springtime change. When it got dark about 8:30, I was out like a light. I awoke about 4 a.m. and was just in and out of sleeping and waking until 7 a.m., when I became aware of the feeling of wanting to dream. I wanted to get to a particular dream as if it was waiting for me. I wondered what I was looking for. I felt there was a dream coming about love. I tried to think about lovers, and nothing compelling came to mind (laughs). No voice said, "That is what or whom you want to dream about."

RM: So you were looking for a dream with a theme of love?

N: Yes, and then, as I woke up, I had a perception of the possibility that on the other side of the great leap, that leap into the next way of being that we've talked about, where we will land, is pure love. Not material, not temporal, not qualitative, just unconditional, absolute love. It's wild. I think that is where we go! (Laughs.)

RM: You have an important, comforting insight, a profound revelation.

Commentary: Nell's revelation could be taken directly from the Bible: "God is love, and whoever abides in love abides in God, and God abides in him" (1 John 4:16).

N: It reminded me of a seminar course on St. Augustine I took in 1979. The professor taught us that Augustine really thought that the universe was sustained in being at every moment by love. That is what God was, love, the motivating force that kept everything going. Not circumscribed by time or matter, certainly not anthropomorphic, but the foundation of everything. Suppose that on the other end of my daring trapeze leap we envision, I land in absolute love? I thought, "Oh, I am ready to go. I am ready." It was quite a realization. You know, we have worked through some enormously painful, personal questions—life history questions—and these three lines of insight have been building on one another to make it possible—really, deeply—not to be afraid.

Commentary: Nell's reflections call to my mind my questions about death. Does individual consciousness survive? Will we have recollections of this world in the next dimension? Is there a next dimension? Are we simply incorporated into the earth as elements? Do we return to where we came from—stardust? After all, everything we cherish will die. Nell's insight into what awaits her on the other side is comforting. I feel that we have reached one of our therapy goals: understanding and accepting death. Arriving here without fear is special. I wonder how long it will last.

RM: Your insights make it possible to proceed without fear, a good place to be.

N: Isn't it wonderful? I can't guarantee you about number three, but it seems like a good possibility.

RM: It's a wonderful possibility. It came in a flash this morning—is that what you're saying?

N: Yes. It was a beautiful morning. Delicate light was hitting the trees, which are starting to show the colors of their leaf buds. The trees were rendered like a watercolor wash—their almost transparent colors—and the light was glowing. I thought, "That's the love in the dream."

RM: It sounds beautiful.

N: It sounds good to me, too. As a survivor, I'm stumbling along here.

RM: You look and sound graceful to me.

N: I'm stumbling. (Laughs.)

RM: Stumbling with a smile and with laughter, with questions, and a lot to teach—you have a gift that you are giving me personally as well as professionally. This will be a pebble that we are tossing into a pond. The pebble will ripple for many people in a book speaking your wisdom. We are preparing its birth.

N: This is an unexpected stage of life. I didn't know there was going to be a second stage of life called *transition* that would take 15 or 16 months to complete, that it would be a time of such healing, a time to bring the things that have been really painful and very, very negative—bring them to a light and look at them and suffer through them and put them away.

RM: You are brave to talk about your painful past.

N: I remember noting markers of where we were in terms of first recognizing the losses of the past, then mourning them, trying to understand the present, and finally, finding new metaphors for dealing with where we were. I owe Mary a profound debt for helping me see this process as an unfolding. It's like an independent stage of life—this wonderful gardening experience of this past year—a stage of resolution and preparation.

Commentary: *Nell is referring to her childhood memories of mistreatment in her family as well as the emotional distance she has felt from Al over the years. She has made peace with her painful family experiences, found comfort in Al's presence, and forgiven him for past shortcomings. Much of this work was done in conversation prior to our recorded sessions and with her friend Mary, who has training in guided imagery, and regularly spoke with Nell from her home in New York City.*

RM: A gardening experience?

N: To me, it is like a garden, a season in the garden. A whole season to bring things together and get peaceful and strong for the next stage. That is the potential of the stage of life that you are working with as a professional. People come to you in this stage of life, and then part of your job is to help them discern its distinct time and its distinct task as a springboard to the future.

RM: You are saying there are possibilities in mortal time—even at the end, you can make new discoveries?

N: Yes, yes! If the sun keeps coming up and sending me such wonderful messages, who knows? It was so beautiful this morning.
It was just lovely.

RM: A message of love, beautiful.

N: Yeah, it was lovely, and the air was so sweet and fresh, and the
birds were just going to town.

RM: The ordinary miracles of the day are available to you because
you are paying attention; you are awake and seeing. When you
reflect on light, air, the sounds of spring outside your window,
experience love, you are reaching for the transcendent. You
are momentarily moving beyond the bounds of your body.

N: Yes, that's what it's like. That's my new information since I last
saw you.

RM: That's big! Phenomenal insights.

N: The answer to the question of "when" is no longer pressing,
and that has a lot to do with this increase in freedom. I feel like
I am already in between worlds or in both—living and dying.
I sleep more. I sleep and wake and sleep and wake in a quasi-
dream-like state. It's preparation, too. It's already happening.

RM: Tell me of your sleep/wake stage.

N: Usually I sleep 12 or 13 hours, and then I wake up, and Sally is
here now four mornings a week. She makes my milkshake. She
came to us through an agency. She does the laundry and keeps
house, does the grocery shopping, keeps the bird feeders full
and the plants watered. She's wonderful, a positive and gentle
spirit. We decided her presence was a priority. She will make
my breakfast, which I have in bed. This is the most delicate
time of the day, waking up the GI tract. Eating can cause so
much pain; it is less severe if I'm reclining and if I take lots of
time. If it takes 30 minutes to drink a milkshake, that's OK.
Then I may doze in and out. I don't know why some days I need
15 hours and some days just 12 or 13. I haven't found anything
that correlates with that sleep need, but I have learned to obey
my body and sleep as it requires! (Laughs.)[4]

RM: You said you had pain when you move about. Is that what you feel now?

N: I definitely do feel it when I move, but I also feel it if I try to sit. The tumor is so large now that it's a burden to sit upright. I mostly conduct business right here in bed and try not to get bedsores.

RM: You're managing well with the medicine and your routine. You're comfortable now?

N: I took a couple of morphine pills shortly before you came. Morphine doesn't knock me out. I am very lucky. It's calming. Apparently, it acts as a muscle relaxant in addition to pain relief. To me, it is soothing.

RM: Well, that's good. It can make people tired.

N: Oh, no! (Laughs.) It makes me very happy.

RM: Good! You're pulling together a transcendent experience as well as managing the tasks of each day. There's activity with the emotional/spiritual part of this stage, and running parallel to that is the mundane—eating, sleeping, managing pain, and the management of everyday life. You are doing both well.

N: Thank you. I keep learning. Over Easter weekend, I had three bouts of vomiting through the night, and I really didn't want to call anybody on a holiday. I thought about calling the ambulance but decided to tough it out. I should have called hospice, but I didn't have that habit—when it's appropriate to call hospice. I didn't call hospice until Monday, but then the LPN came over, and she introduced me to Compazine, which was very effective. I've been able to keep food down ever since.

Commentary: Managing physical symptoms of the disease and its treatment is an art and science. The task is to match the symptom with a medication and/or a behavioral/psychological technique. For example, nausea can be managed by many medications, some with side effects that are equally troubling to patients. Thus, it becomes a trial-and-error effort, where good provider–patient communication is essential for optimal management. Simple breathing and guided-imagery and mindfulness exercises can also help reduce nausea. Most newly diagnosed patients treated for the first time on chemo-therapy go through a learning curve, understanding what they can expect from the medication and what symptoms can be treated. Often this involves a rethinking of what it means to "complain." Describing symptoms is not complaining; it is being a good patient and helping the healthcare team address the symptom. All healthcare providers have an obligation and responsibility to help the patient manage symptoms with whatever tools that are available, including education and advocacy.

RM: That's great. You are having experiences with symptoms—mundane, worldly—and with themes, particularly with the experience of a leap to love. That is transcendent. You've got your feet in two different worlds.

N: Yes, I do feel like that. I feel like I'm just going to slip over.

RM: Well, yes. You're opening yourself to the other side. Your head and your heart are open to the movement. I see you've got the book by John O'Donohue with the idea that the horizon is in the well.[5]

N: That's right. His work is rich with useful metaphors, and his writing is like poetry.

RM: Have you chosen, or do you have, any spiritual ushers like Fr. O'Donohue for this journey? Priests, clergy that you know that you want to perform the Anointing of the Sick?

N: Fr. Bob has given me the Anointing of the Sick twice. He is very generous. He anointed Al, too. But I was disappointed in the sacrament. Not being a cradle Catholic, what do I know about last rites?[6] But I read this wonderful book last summer, *A Mass for the Dead*, by the playwright William Gibson, that gave me a picture of the process.[7] Gibson was raised Catholic, although even as a child he did not assent to its religious principles. His father was Protestant by heritage but not practicing. They lived in a close-knit, hard-working, very Irish, very Catholic neighborhood on the northernmost tip of Manhattan. The book is a panegyric to his parents and an exploration of his own formation. The book ends as his mother receives last rites and dies. His description of the sacrament was powerful to me because of the way it addressed the body as well as the spirit. Let me read to you:

> "I watched the priest at the candle moisten his thumb in holy oil. With the sign of the cross, he anointed her eyelids, praying aloud for forgiveness for the wrong she had done by the use of her sight, dipped his thumb and anointed her ears, praying for forgiveness for the wrong she had done by the use of her hearing. Dipped his thumb to anoint her nostrils, and I saw he was purging her body of the deeds of its senses. It was a rite that for 1000 years had made peace with the defects of the human material, and the thumb of the priest anointed her mouth for the wrongs of its taste and speech, and her open palms, for touch, and lastly her feet for the wrong done by her power to walk."

RM: That is powerful.

N: Liturgically, this cleansing of the body, the absolution of its history, was set within a familiar frame of ancient prayers. I was knocked out by the concreteness of the rite's recognition that it is in our bodies that we live. And of course it is in our bodies that we die. So I looked forward to my anointing, thinking it would be the same. When Fr. Bob asked if I wanted to be anointed, I said, "Yes! Do I get all the senses?" And he said, "No, we don't do that anymore. We have a shortened version," and I was so let down.

RM: Well, I guess that means that some of the organs you've sinned with haven't quite cleared inspection then. (Both laugh.)

N: Sometimes I think the church does not understand the trans-verbal, the trans-noetic dimensions it is working with. It streamlines too much. We already have what we need in the liturgy, but we need to understand it better and nurture it. To take away the senses—how dumb is that!?

RM: Yes, it does seem peculiar. Now, I want to switch gears and ask you about what you said the last time we spoke—that the table was clear, and you had no duties left to perform, and yet you felt caught in the world because you had so many interests. Now, it seems, you are in a different place?

N: I was afraid that I didn't know when to turn off the fighter en-gine. There is a time when one should stop performing. If the analogy is about flying, I should be prepared to glide like the swan to transition out.[8] (Box 3.1) I'm not anxious anymore

---

Box 3.1 The Swan

Rainer Maria Rilke

> This laboring of ours with all that remains undone,
> as if still bound to it,
> is like the lumbering gait of the swan.
> And then our dying—releasing ourselves
> from the very ground on which we stood—
> is like the way he hesitantly lowers himself
> into the water. It gently receives him
> and, gladly yielding, flows back beneath him,
> as wave follows wave,
> while he, now wholly serene and sure,
> with regal composure,
> allows himself to glide.

about being engaged or not being engaged. I think that's part of the freedom that came with the second realization we talked about earlier. I'm not worried about going, so I'm not worried about staying.

RM: Wise.

N: And I am much more comfortable.

RM: Looks like you might be able to take a little nap now? Are you fading?

N: I'm starting to fade.

RM: I have a poem by Franz Wright called "On Earth."[9] You will recognize part of this from our earlier conversations.

N: Please read it (Box 3.2).

N: Yes, that is nice.

Box 3.2 On Earth

Franz Wright

Resurrection of the little apple tree outside
my window, leaf-
light of late
in the April
called her eyes, forget
forget—
but how
How does one go about dying?
Who on earth
is going to teach me—
The world
is filled with people
who have never died

RM: And so we come to think about that phrase, "for those who have never died," and our conversation, this co-creation through our meetings. We are bringing something into the world. Our conversation is for those who have never died.

N: That is wonderful.

Final Commentary: *Nell's ruminations about the Catholic faith stir my own spiritual inclinations as a cradle Catholic born into a conservative Irish Catholic family in Peoria, IL, raised as a child and adolescent on doctrine, and in my adulthood "fitfully Catholic." I am not unlike Nell, wondering at times even while singing in the choir: Do I belong in my own church? Such questions have emerged for me on this journey with Nell.*

Franz Wright's poem is an eloquent call for a teacher about death. "How does one go about dying? Who on earth is going to teach me?" I have come to see Nell as my teacher, as she sees me as her companion on the road. The question posed in this poem has followed me throughout my professional career in cancer care: How does one go about dying? In our first meeting, Nell asked this same question. As you will see later, her answer emerges in our dialogues over time as she finally arrives home even while preparing to depart this earth.

Notes

1. McQuellon, R. P., & Cowan, M. A. (2000). Turning toward death together: Conversation in mortal time. *American Journal of Hospice & Palliative Care, 17*(5), 312–318.

2. Nell is referring to making peace with her family history of mistreatment, Al's emotional distance over the years, and the painful reality of his slow decline due to Alzheimer's disease.

3. Atul Gawande, author of *Being Mortal*, lists five end-of-life questions for patients to consider. They have appeared in various forms similar to the following: (1) What is your understanding of where you are and of your illness? (2) What are your fears or worries for the future? (3) What are goals and priorities? (4) What outcomes are unacceptable to you? What are you

willing to sacrifice and not? (5) And later, what would a good day look like? See Campbell, S. (2015, February 10). Atul Gawande's 5 questions to ask at life's end. *Next Avenue: Caregiving*. https://www.nextavenue.org/atul-gawandes-5-questions-ask-lifes-end

4. Nell's approach is like that of the Zen masters. When asked by his student, "Master, how do you practice Zen?" he replied, "When you are hungry, eat; when you are tired, sleep." http://www.sinc.sunysb.edu/Clubs/buddhism/story/story.html

5. O'Donohue, J. (1997). *Anam cara*. New York: Harper. Chapter 6, "Death: The horizon is in the well," begins:

> There is a presence who walks the road of life with you. This presence accompanies your every moment. It shadows your every thought and feeling. On your own, or with others, it is always there with you. When you were born, it came out of the womb with you; with the excitement at your arrival, nobody noticed it. Though this presence surrounds you, you may still be blind to its companionship. The name of this presence is death. (p. 199)

6. The term *last rites* refers to the sacraments that Catholics receive at the end of their lives; specifically, Confession, Holy Communion, and the Anointing of the Sick, and the prayers accompanying each. The phrase is less common today than in past centuries. While last rites sometimes refer to only one of the seven sacraments, the Sacrament of the Anointing of the Sick (also known as the Sacrament of the Sick), that application is technically incorrect. The Sacrament of the Anointing of the Sick, previously known as Extreme Unction, is administered to both the dying and those who are gravely ill or about to undergo a serious operation to pray for the recovery of their health and spiritual strength. The Anointing of the Sick is technically part of the last rites rather than the last rite itself.

7. Gibson, W. (1968). *A mass for the dead*. New York: Atheneum.

8. In one of our meetings before we began recording, I gave Nell the poem "The Swan" by Rainer Maria Rilke (Box 3.2).

9. Wright, F. (2004). "On earth." In *Walking to Martha's Vineyard*. New York: Alfred A. Knopf.

4

April 12, 2005—Letting Go and Mastering Fear

When you practice looking deeply,
you see your true nature of no birth, no death;
no being, no non-being;
no going, no same no different.
When you see this you are free from fear

> Hanh, T. N. (2002). *No death, no fear: Comforting
> wisdom for life* (p. 63). New York: Riverhead Books.

Main Themes: Mastering fear and letting go of worldly anchoring activities.

At our last meeting, Nell felt that death was coming soon and welcomed the prospect. Today, she speaks of managing her difficult breathing and letting go of the activities that grounded her in this life. She finds comfort in the simple pleasure of watching a TV program with spouse Al and beloved cat Amber curled up beside her. It distracts her from the fear that moves through her when she feels short of breath and contemplates dying.

I have told Nell about our group of psychosocial oncology providers in the cancer patient support program I direct at Wake Forest Baptist Health. Gail Hurt has both nursing and counseling degrees and has expressed a special interest in Nell when I speak of her at our weekly administrative/supervisory meetings. Gail has been my dear colleague and companion in Nell's care, providing poems and other reference materials that relate to our dialogues. She gave me the poem that I brought today.

Nell is adapting to daily physical deterioration. Managing changing bodily functions often requires using medication and behavioral changes to solve a problem from the first time it appears, which calls for close work with healthcare providers. We begin with her most pressing concern: fear of suffocating.

Dialogue 4

N: I learned something this week. My problem right now is breathing. I called hospice and said, "I give up. Send me some oxygen!"

RM: OK, good call.

N: Yes. It's just that they ask peculiar questions like, "Do you have any appetite?" when I'm asking for air! I have an enormous appetite. I just have no place to put it! It's the same as breathing. I love to breathe; I just have no place to breathe with this tumor taking space. It's hard to get comfortable.

RM: This is a very good decision. When you get the nasal cannula, you won't have to breathe so deeply, and you'll still get more oxygen. You will have to cut down on cigar smoking here. (Both laugh.)

N: Our friend Kristin called this afternoon. She had gone to her aunt, who is the secretary at the church. She got a vigil candle because it will burn seven days straight.

RM: Uh-oh—not with oxygen here.

N: I declined. I wouldn't have a candle here, even without oxygen, not without an attendant. I just feel too responsible, being in this apartment building. We could set the place on fire. We are all pretty infirm, so I said thank you, but no thanks.

RM: Good thinking.

N: I had oxygen at home in October, but they wanted me to carry it around with me and all that. I was very resistant and rebellious. I did not want it, but now it's OK.

RM: You'll think more clearly, and it won't take so much energy to breathe.

N: I'm getting discouraged about this dying process.

RM: Discouraged and yet there's a smile on your face.

Commentary: *Nell typically comments about harsh realities with a smile. Calling attention to this apparent incongruity is my way of encouraging her to explore how she feels about the very serious topic of her own dying.*

N: Well, I hope to stay smiling. What I learned this week is I don't need to worry about figuring out the timeline because the tumor is here. I left the tumor out of the count. We've been talking all this time about mind and body, and yet there's a third reality. The third reality is neither me nor not me—it's the damn tumor! (Laughs.) And the damn tumor has a life of its own. It's parasitic on mine but quite different from mine. It's pretty much calling the shots. I can observe that now more than anyone. I'm not so much in doubt about how much longer I have. I do very much feel that I'm in the "leap range."[1] Even with Anna, who I love so much and who is so sensitive and gentle, I can't be up and be present to her for more than a little while. Now I don't really care if the paper comes or doesn't come. It was my little totem—getting the daily *New York Times* and reading it—my ritual. But my ritual of being here is going away. I think I'm fading, like Tinker Bell.

Commentary: *When Nell speaks of her own death humorously and identifies the tumor as having a life of its own, it surprises me. She does it while at the same time acknowledging letting go of her activities, the simple things that occupy much of her time and anchor her to the world. She is describing loss; grief is the companion of loss, but*

I don't see it now. So far, sadness has not been a frequent visitor to our conversations. I wonder if I should encourage Nell to speak of her grief now. I settle for a general question about fading.

RM: What is coming to you when you're fading?

N: It's been very beautiful except when I'm struggling to breathe. That's what I was describing to you last week when I looked out the window. It's the air, the color and the smell of the air, the life. I normally sleep now 13 or 14 hours. When I wake up, it will be the middle of the day sometimes. On rainy days, like the last few days, I see a kind of opalescent beautiful shimmery light in my room—it's more of a feeling. I remember there was a time when I was still harvesting imagery, conversations, events, friendships, and travels. That doesn't seem to matter much anymore. It's just a very quiet time. I come in and out of sleeping.

RM: Coming in and out of sleeping on no particular schedule is OK?

N: Unless there's basketball or baseball on TV. (Laughs.) We do have this evening ritual where we will watch one thing on television. That is our nightly ritual. I get up, and I have pillows that I put on the floor, and I lie on the floor with Amber beside me. Al sits on the couch, and we watch. Usually Amber competes for attention when there's company.[2]

RM: You and Amber and Al all watching the tube.

N: Amber curls up beside me, and we watch the tube. We are right in front of the TV, and Al's on the couch. We rent from Netflix—they're usually shorter than a movie—sometimes one-hour segments, sometimes more. Yesterday, since there were so many televised sports for his majesty Al to watch (laughs), I did a *Sopranos* marathon. I did four hours of *The Sopranos*.[3]

RM: You were awake for four hours straight watching *The Sopranos*!?

N: Not straight, I broke it up. That was kind of fun. I've only seen two seasons now, but I've become very attached to the Sopranos.

RM: Have you now?

N: I've decided that they are exactly like us. That's the revelation. Number one: Each one of us has the potential to be really spoiled, which is what they are. They are just out-of-control spoiled. They just do it with guns. You know? We do it otherwise, but they have no impulse control. As Tony said once to his nephew, "Impulse control—that's what he needs to learn." Tony decides when he is going to kill somebody; other people do it impulsively. (Laughs.) So it's that dimension of ourselves that we edit out so rigorously, and then there is the common humanity, which mostly gets expressed by the women much of the time. Lately, it's also gradually, bit by bit, layers are sort of coming off, and you see the men struggling with relational sensitivity and bonds or closeness that are very important to them. I find it sort of like visiting Mars (laughs) and finding out that these characters look really different from us, but inside we're all the same. I'm enjoying it a lot.

RM: Well, that's nice. Some things are falling away, like the newspaper and the daily rituals, and yet there are moments and even hours like watching *The Sopranos* or watching a basketball game together with Al that are just fine. And there is a real unusual sense of humor in these TV episodes as well as insights about human beings?

N: Oh, yes, funny and powerful.

RM: I can see your energy and animation from watching these peculiar characters come to life. This is less taxing on your energy than reading. Books like *Arresting God in Kathmandu*[4] are a little bit more than what you need right now or want right now?

N: If there were another *Arresting God in Kathmandu*, that would be great. It's not often that a book like that falls into one's lap. It's on a par with *The Kite Runner*. Did we talk about *The Kite Runner*?[5]

RM: We didn't. Did you like it?

N: I liked it much more intensely than Al did. Al liked it, but I really, really like it. The author is from Afghanistan. I think part of the attraction for me was I have never been there. Al's been to all of these places.

RM: So he has more of a connection to these places.

N: Yes. In a sense, it's not all new to him. To me, it's a kind of point of entry into a Third World. I went all of my life without encountering the Third World really, and it's most of the world.

RM: Yes, I see. Now, let me ask you a couple of questions about practical things. The oxygen is a good idea. You haven't liked the use of oxygen in the past, but you've come to accept it now. It's going to come to you tomorrow?

N: I don't know. Have you ever dealt with hospice? You have to go through a phone tree, so I left a voice message. It may take a few days to get the voice message through. The line is always busy. Three or four times when I call the main number, it's busy, and then I call the fallback number. It takes a lot of effort. It's partly that they don't have the people to man the phones, so they just put them on hold.

Commentary: I changed the topic from The Kite Runner *to address Nell's shortness of breath. My primary agenda is to hear what's on her mind. And, as her patient-advocate, I want to assure that her symptoms are managed well.*

Therapists sometimes make the arbitrary distinction between shooting the breeze/elevator talk—for example, discussing The Kite Runner*—and psychotherapy, often a difference without merit, since the manifest content may convey deeper meaning on further scrutiny. Nell's reflections on* The Kite Runner *and* The Sopranos *are a window into her thoughtful analysis of literature and television. Discussion of* The Kite Runner *is a way to think about the differences between her and Al.* The Sopranos *offers the opportunity to study human nature. Nell concludes that we are all very similar, reminding me of psychiatrist Harry Stack Sullivan's axiom, "We are all much more simply human than otherwise, be we happy and successful, contented and detached, miserable and mentally disordered."[6] The idea of a common* *bond in the human community, a sense of us rather than "them", is an enduring value of Nell's.*

The topics we discuss cannot revolve solely around death. The emotional intensity of death talk cannot be sustained over long periods. The death journey must be leavened by discussing the ordinary events of the day. "Ordinary conversation" is important and full of meaning. Nell has described the breeze through her window after a spring rain, the brilliant sunset, cardinals singing —these wonders of the day give life meaning. As her therapist, my duty is to guide the conversation while not controlling it. Therapeutic conversation is like a dance where the partners take turns leading and following.

RM: So the message is in—no call back yet?

N: No.

RM: It's good that you got the message in. You also have some discomfort, and you took a pill. Is it helping?

N: I took it just before you came, and it is helping already. The medication is consistent. I take four different pills for the sake of different things. It used to be more explicit pain, like stabbing pain, and now it's a duller pain, an intense feeling of being crushed.

RM: It's the tumor growing. Did the hospice nurse check you this week?

N: The nurse came yesterday. She felt the tumor had increased. The LPN came today, and she just did the abdomen, not the tumor area. That was because I was practically asleep. I just could not wake up enough, and she did not want to be intrusive, so she went away, which was sweet of her. I am using the Compazine for nausea, and that helps. Otherwise, I don't know what I would do. Remember your mental fantasy about stopping eating? You thought you might just stop eating, or you could stop drinking in order to die? The harder it is to eat, the hungrier I feel!

RM: So my tale about how I might leave this world if faced with my ending was just that—a fantasy? (Laughs.)

N: Well, for me, it would be a fantasy. I'm too appetitive, I guess. (Laughs.)

RM: You're hungry?

N: Yes. Apparently what Compazine does is relax those muscles to help move things along, so that food doesn't get all stacked up there, and I start choking.

RM: You're doing a great job with the mechanics of body management—air, food, comforts.

N: This is what's so scary, Dick. It's good to have a positive attitude, blah, blah, blah. But this is closing down on me, and I'm scared of what it's going to feel like. I understand now why they dope people at the end, and they're welcome to dope me up. I don't want to feel like I'm choking to death. That's an experience I can forgo.

Commentary: Nell reacts to my compliment about how well she is doing. She is very polite and does not contradict me directly, rather saying "blah, blah, blah." I think she is gently telling me that my encouragement and "you are doing a great job" are missing how hard life is getting for her. I try to remain positive and yet allow room for the sadness, grief, and anger that are often just below the surface when the unfairness of cancer is experienced and named. Some patients are off-put by too much "false positive chatter", sometimes referred to as "brightsiding", when a caregiver exhorts them to be optimistic, harping too much on the positive without acknowledging the darkness that accompanies life threatening illness. There is a delicate balance between hollow positivity and affirmative presence, requiring good judgment honed by experience.

As Nell's body deteriorates, her perspective on being heavily medicated changes. Earlier, she said, "I do not want to be doped up and miss the transition." Her shifting perspective reminds me of a quote I saw on our hospital's medical oncology unit: "Blessed are the flexible, for they shall never be bent out of shape." Nell is demonstrating her flexibility by changing her hopes and plans for her death. The prospect of medication at the end is now acceptable. Always have a Plan B.

RM: I am with you. I will be here if you need me to help avoid that situation. All right? You have my numbers—home phone, cell phone, work phone—just to make sure that if you need immediate care, I can help you make it happen. OK?

N: Thank you.

RM: It's important to be protected from that feeling of being crushed. It may never come to that, but it's good to have insurance.

N: I hope it doesn't come to that. (Sighs.) Being crushed—that's exactly what it feels like.

RM: To be free from anxiety and worry about physical symptoms is to allow the simple pleasures to continue. Looking out your window at the landscape and the cardinals, having that insight of leaping to love at the end. It's very hard to pay attention to much of anything if you are in pain. I keep saying, you are managing the mechanics of the body well, even though you do have occasional problems. Who knows how to do this for the first time? Hospice nurses and docs have a good idea. You are learning and taking action when necessary. You made a good decision to bring in hospice. They have done better recently than they did on the first run. It's important to have a lifeline.

N: Yes. I think the trick there was keeping Dr. T, you, and the clinic in the loop. Just building that buffer was the crucial thing. I also asked on the voicemail for them to get their ducks in a row. I'm supposed to go to the clinic next week to see Dr. T. I have blood work and will get the port-a-catheter flushed.[7] Hospice could do everything, but I want to see Dr. T. It's just a hospice courtesy policy to work with Dr. T.

Commentary: I am volunteering to be one more person on call for Nell, knowing that she has her medical team as the first line. I am extending the boundaries of intervention by giving out my home and cell phone numbers. Providing a lifeline eventually proves very useful when Nell has a panic-like attack after an upsetting exchange with one of her professional caregivers.

RM: OK. Dr. T is the best. Now we are coming to the end of our time. I want to make sure we've covered all bases. Is there anything else on your mind, in your heart, you want to talk about?

N: I would love to see the transcript for our last meeting when it is available

RM: OK. I will email it tomorrow.

N: That would be so terrific. I would like to see it because there were a few things that I said there that I would like to clarify.

RM: What you said was fine, and anything you want to clarify is fine, but I don't want this to become a demanding editorial task for you.

N: Well, I realize that I am not capable of doing a huge editorial task. I look, I read it all, and I realize that it's a lot. Did I ever tell you that I used to edit for Studs Terkel?

RM: No kidding!

N: Those big interview books that he did. Actually, I know a fair amount about editing interviews, but I do not have the energy to even approach this very rambly stuff. But I wondered how you envision using it?

RM: One way to use our transcript would be to have an introductory statement and comments from me about parts of our dialogue. This may become a small book, pamphlet, or article. Rest assured that your story and you will remain in my head and heart for a long time, and our story will be heard.

N: Yes, OK. And I hope you live a long time, and I would love to be an animator in some way! Thank you.

RM: You're welcome. Thank you. OK. So with mechanics you are doing well—with transcendence, doing great.

N: Pretty good. Hanging in there.

RM: I have something I want to read to you before I leave.

N: OK.

RM: This is a poem given to me by my colleague Gail Hurt (Box 4.1).

N: Oh, yes, I remember Gail.

Box 4.1 You Were Born

Rabindranath Tagore

You were born to the joy of all
the blue sky,
birds
your mother's eyes;
Sravan's rains, *sarat's* moist air,
these were the first welcome of life.
Your birth was given in an instant
an endless gift,
the call of home to the home-dweller.

Death be yours in distant loneliness at night
greet you where sea-waves rhythm the dance of the homeless,
where a chant rises from the unknown forest,
where the foreign waterfall claps its hands in a farewell song,
where unfamiliar stars offer light to the infinite,
where nothing calls back to return.
The door is open: Oceans and hills all point to the road.
The night near your head will stand silent
For death is a call to the wayfarer.[8]

RM: Gail said, "I thought of Nell when I read this." I want to read this to you and see what you think. It has elements of the transcendent.

N: Yes, please read it.

N: Wonderful. "Death is a call to the wayfarer." There is a line I wrote down somewhere, and I've lost it. It was very like that. Death calls to me. There must be a synergy in reading these things together. Thank you.

RM: You're welcome. And I thank you.

N: I'm so scared. It's just the unknown of it. But it would be crazy not to be scared. Well, almost crazy. It would be blessed not to be scared.

Commentary: When Nell said, "I'm so scared," it took me aback and elicited my own fear for her. I feel her fear and share it. I know from experience that crafting a good death requires competence, a good team, and luck at the end. Even as she expresses her fear, she comforts herself with a chuckle, noting that not being scared would be a blessing. Nell does not stay long in fear. I hope naming her feelings will help to calm her fear now. I hope I can help her to avoid a fear-filled death in the end. I agree that to die without fear would be a blessing.

RM: Yes, it would. There are times when you move into fear, and other times when you are very peaceful.

N: The times when I move into fear are times when I've been in touch with physical discomfort. It's the physical.

RM: That makes sense.

N: After telling you the tumor is an independent force, that there is a third character in this story, I considered this: There is a qualitative difference between the experience of terminal cancer when you can see and feel your tumor and when you can't, like [with] lung cancer, when you can't see it. I would think that would be two very different experiences of dying. Just being in daily communication with this thing that clearly has its own mind, as it were, or non-mind is an education. That's the whole problem. There is no impulse control for the tumor! (Laughs.)

Commentary: This insight regarding the difference between the cancer you can see and the cancer you can't see is important. Cancer patients with visible evidence of their disease may be treated differently than those with an "invisible" tumor. Specifically, the visible results of cancer or its treatment—for example, disfiguring surgery—may allow patients to be excused from daily household tasks. Also, the reality of a visible, palpable tumor brings home to the patient and caregiver the relentless movement of the disease. Nell is also right about cancer's lack of impulse control; cancer cells have no shut-off valve to slow their relentless growth.

RM: No impulse control? Better turn this tumor over to Tony Soprano, then!

N: Yes (hearty laugh).

RM: (Laughs.) Do you need anything before I leave?

N: No. I'm OK.

RM: Between now and then, if anything comes up—if you need an advocate, and you don't want to put it all on Al—call me. I will be accessible.

N: Yes, OK. I could use a hug.

RM: I could give one.

N: (Chuckles.) I thank you so much.

RM: (Nell's tears flow as I hug her. We pause for minute.) Those tears are healing.

N: I thank you for a good hug.

RM: You're very welcome.

Final Commentary: *Nell's tears are a sign of good grief. She is letting go and gets relief from her tears, a sign that they are healing, not that she is clinically depressed. While much of our conversation is punctuated by laughter, there are periods of deep sadness. I am glad that Nell trusts me enough to ask for a hug. Often her tears come as she reflects on the losses in her life—little losses and the ultimate loss on the horizon, her own life and all that she holds dear.*

By managing her physical problems and symptoms, Nell can engage in her important everyday activities, stitched together to make meaning. I have responsibility for helping her to identify her symptoms and to communicate them to the medical team, so they may be able to address them. Some patients ignore symptoms or fail to state them with enough force to get attention, and consequently, they do not get effective treatment.

For Nell, this experience is once in a lifetime. For the medical team, it is an everyday event. That difference can lead to a failed empathic connection and an inadequate response to symptoms. Nell was feeling disconnected from her hospice team. She did not feel they were tending to her needs with a sense of urgency. I want to be useful to Nell but not overstep my role by intervening. Am I doing enough?

Notes

1. Nell and I often spoke of death as the "great leap to another dimension."
2. An important player in Nell's story is her beloved cat Amber. While he may appear only several times in the dialogues, he was a constant presence and source of tactile comfort for her, snuggling on the bed. His presence became increasingly important as she deteriorated physically and became thinner and weaker. She would often be stroking him when she spoke with me, and he would purr with delight.
3. *The Sopranos* was a television series broadcast from 1999 to 2007. The story includes therapy sessions between a psychiatrist and a mobster.
4. Upadhyay, S. (2001). *Arresting God in Kathmandu*. Boston: Houghton Mifflin.
5. Hosseini, K. (2003). *The kite runner*. New York: Riverhead Books.
6. Sullivan, H. S. (1966). *Conceptions of modern psychiatry* (p. 7). New York: W. W. Norton and Company, Inc.
7. A port-a-catheter is a device used to diminish patient discomfort when chemotherapy treatments, intravenous fluids, drugs, or blood transfusions must be delivered frequently. The port is placed under the skin, usually in the chest just over the breast area. It is attached to a thin, flexible tube (the catheter), which is guided, or threaded, into the superior vena cava, a large vein above the right side of the heart. A needle can then be inserted into the port to draw blood or to give fluids.
8. Chakravarty, A. (Ed.) (1966). *A Tagore reader* (p. 351). Boston: Beacon Press.

5

April 19, 2005—Leaving Gifts

Feelings come and go like clouds in a windy sky. Conscious
breathing is my anchor.

Hanh, T. N. (2001). *Stepping into freedom:*
Rules of monastic practice for novices.
Berkeley: Parallax Press.

Main Themes: Giving gifts, letting go, the problem of self-advocacy,
and confronting the fear of suffocation—"like skating in the dark."
Nell is grateful for her medical oncologist, who has continued
to manage her pain medication through hospice. This unusual
arrangement works well. Generally, the hospice medical team
manages medication because they have eyes on the patient regularly. There was a problem with getting her oxygen set up properly,
which led to additional problems. We used a simple breathing exercise to quiet the panic that arises with the feeling of suffocation.
Nell has been giving her possessions away to friends and relatives.
She is generous and wants to shed her worldly objects and leave
something behind for special people in her life. She is delighted to
have discovered a way of giving that can help her niece with her
summer plans. She begins with this good news.

Dialogue 5

N: I have some good news to tell you—the most wonderful news.
Suddenly, I got this idea Thursday night on the floor watching

TV. See that picture on the wall there? Those two neat kids are the two children of my oldest nephew.

RM: Yes, I see big kids. Tell me the good news.

N: Their parents are tall, and they are very athletic. Their father is in the Coast Guard, and their mom is a full-time mother. They have made some economic decisions about parenting and how and what matters. She comes from northern Michigan. They are always posted far from home, and every summer she goes with the kids to Michigan and spends quality time with their grandparents and cousins. This year, they've had car trouble, and gas prices are really hitting them. For working people, they're hitting much harder than we realize. Most of us can swallow the gas price increases without hurting, but for many people, it's a real budget item. This all came up because she sent me some funny, darling pictures of cakes she has been baking. She has a website that she runs from home, and the money from it is designated for the summer trip to Traverse City, Michigan, from Seattle.

RM: Big trip.

N: Big trip, expensive trip. Well, the little genie that walks through my head, so excited, said, "Why not use the frequent-flyer miles for them?" It took two days, and by Saturday morning, we had it done—got the tickets, all with frequent-flyer miles. I needed 120,000 miles. I had 121! (Both laugh.)

RM: Beautiful!

N: (Laughs.) I thought, this is the ultimate salvage. I have been trying to find for each person I've cared about just the right gift —things of mine that I knew people liked. But this was really beyond my imagination.

RM: It's a wonderful gift. It must have taken some work to get it done.

N: It *did* take work because frequent-flyer miles are getting harder and harder to redeem. If Carla, my niece by marriage, had not been so good at the computer, we would not have gotten the fourth ticket because their agent couldn't find the ticket for Jeff. She just went in there and drilled out through the system. Jeff is in Florida right now doing some HAZMAT training, and she has the kids alone. She was being mom and dad at Little League Friday night, and she took her laptop with her and found the missing link, which was taking a red eye via Dallas. It worked! I was on cloud nine for three days. I just had to get back there to cloud nine.

RM: That is very good news indeed.

N: It was exciting. Now I know that they'll be having all that pleasure this summer. I will just look down from the heavens, eying them in Michigan. It's Traverse City, Michigan. Very, very, very pretty.

Commentary: *The theme of letting go and giving away objects has developed in our conversations. Nell is pleased to give this trip to her nephew and his family. Her generosity, giving away her worldly possessions, will make a difference for someone else. Telling me her frequent-flyer miles adventure lifts her spirits and mine. What better way to give meaning to the day?*

RM: Excellent. Now, have you heard from your sister Ruth?

N: Oh, every few days. They're still getting battered and hammered, quite bad fortune, but her husband got out of the hospital after a week, and they're just taking it a day at a time. They have not succeeded in selling their truck. That leaves them with two options. One is to get back on the road and drive the truck until it's paid for, which is five more years. The other is to declare bankruptcy. They are not good options. I don't understand why they couldn't just sell the truck at some horrendous loss but get out from under it. It's an 18-wheeler.

RM: They have some things to work on, to try to figure out. You said there was some positive and negative news?

N: Remember Tuesday? The wonderful celerity with which hospice sent over the oxygen machine?

RM: Yes, that was impressive.

N: That was impressive, but they didn't have a humidifier for it, so by Friday, I was having constant nosebleeds. I called Friday and said, "I am on 6 milligrams of Coumadin, and I'm having constant nosebleeds. I think I need help here." They said, "Yes, you do. You need a humidifier. We'll get right on it." Guess what "get right on it" meant? It came today—four days later! They are just empty plastic bottles tailored to that particular machine. "We'll get right on it!" If you're not mad yet, you're going to get mad!

RM: I am getting there.

N: Well, I was too. I called Friday again. Monday, I called three times. Monday, they said they had ordered the bottle, and it would be delivered. They were going to be delivered Monday or Tuesday. And I said, "That's hunky-dory—whatever it is you're sending me, what am I going to do with it?" They said, "Don't you have a nurse there?" Duh. If I had a nurse here, would I care about hospice? I would not call them ever, and I barked, "No, I don't have a nurse here!"

RM: You are getting really annoyed with them at this point. It doesn't sound like you.

N: I managed not to get sarcastic and not to lose my temper at any time, but I was not my usual warm, mature self. I called them three times on Monday and just got the runaround, and I explained that I did not have a nurse on the premises. "Well, then," they said, "we'll need to send somebody to hook this up for you and show you how it works." I said, "Yes, you will, but since it isn't here, there isn't much to talk about!" Things kind of spiraled downward from there.

RM: A very unsatisfactory call.

N: Yes, well, Anna was here. I was so dry that I couldn't swallow, and I kept swallowing and started suffocating. The mucous membranes just would not let me swallow. I was getting that choking feeling. The only thing that would help would be to sit upright and take a drink of water. I was like a baby. I kind of burped back, and that would get the swallow to happen. I was beside myself last night. I had called three times on Monday.

RM: The oxygen came a week ago, but the humidifier didn't come until—?

N: I'll tell you when the humidifier came—Monday, last night about 9 o'clock! I was really starting to panic. I called hospice and said I was not willing to sit up all night waiting to choke, and I needed them to do something now, this evening, right away. Well, they did not think they could do that tonight, blah, blah, blah. She said, "It really has to happen tonight? Well, I could send a nurse out, and she could do that." I said, "Good that's wonderful!"

RM: Yes.

N: Fifteen or 20 minutes later, this nurse calls back. Meanwhile, I'm chugalugging water and getting more panicked, and the nurse said she would need to go out to hospice and pick one up and come over here; she'd be here in about half an hour. It was 10:00 o'clock when she got here last night with the humidifier and hooked it up in five minutes. She was a perfectly terrific nurse! I know her. She works the swing shift at Baptist [Hospital] in Oncology. She is a really nice nurse, and she remembered me. It was a very pleasant meeting. It took an hour or so to calm down enough to sleep. I slept very soundly until hospice woke me up with a call at 8:00 o'clock in the morning to say, "Have you gotten your humidifier yet?" I said I actually was sleeping! (Laughs.)

RM: What a story!

N: Well, I'm mad. I want you tell Dr. T, please. He said to tell him if things like this happen, and if you don't mind just tracking him down? It just should not have happened.

RM: I will put it in writing to him. Let me see if I understand this: When I was here, last Tuesday, you had called and asked for the oxygen. Subsequently, Al took the call from hospice, and the oxygen came out Tuesday night without a humidifier. Then you started having nosebleeds.

N: Yep.

RM: I talked to Al about that last week—I think it was Thursday or Friday. My understanding from him was that you had the humidifier. He told me that you had nosebleeds. I thought he said the humidifier was helping, but maybe he said it was going to help?

N: He must have. Al always wants to minimize difficulties. I always want to solve them. It's not oppositional. It is just a very different way of relating to things, and since people have always solved things for him, it works for him. It does not work for me. If I do not call hospice, my problem does not get solved.

Commentary: Nell is angry with hospice because they have not provided her with all the necessary equipment for the oxygen machine. She is becoming more dependent on others and, for the first time, directly asks me for help, a milestone. She is fiercely independent. I have confidence in hospice and am surprised and puzzled by this glitch. It underscores the bureaucratic hurdles for patients and caregivers who try to manage symptoms with healthcare providers working in different institutions. Engagement across providers and agencies always complicates communication at a time when patients and their family caregivers may not have the energy or know-how to navigate a situation like this.

RM: I missed something because I thought it was solved. I left thinking, "Isn't that great because hospice called back and were coming out that night!" You've taught me the oxygen machine should never be delivered without a humidifier!

N: I told the woman at hospice I had oxygen in October, and they used a different company to deliver the oxygen equipment. It was an entirely different experience. They brought the oxygen and humidifier. They paced out the whole apartment and made sure that I had enough oxygen tubing to go anywhere in the apartment, which I do not have now. They were thoughtful and considerate of me.

RM: Do you want more tubing?

N: There's probably some in the box out in the hall. I just take this nasal cannula off when I need to go into the far corners of Al's world. It's just the thoughtfulness. In other words, it's not the tubing part that's really the problem.

Commentary: *Nell identifies a simple truth in cancer care: Patients want to be listened to and cared for. It's not so much about the tubing; it's about compassionate care demonstrated by consideration and listening. How is a patient using oxygen for the first time to anticipate the need for extra tubing?*

RM: I can tell your energy level is so much different than it was last week.

N: Good or bad?

RM: Good. You were tuckered out last week. I attributed that partly to oxygen deprivation and low hemoglobin. You're a great deal more energetic now. Do you feel that way?

N: Yes, I am, and I just need your help. I need your help on something very specific.

RM: OK.

N: I know it's irrational, but I panic about sleeping. The scary experience yesterday evening was so powerful. I had to sit up in order to swallow; even though it was then followed by a very successful sleep, it just left me without any confidence. I do not want to suffocate. They promised that I would not die of suffocation. I want you to help me down off the panic, to help me off the ledge. Is there a way to do that?

RM: Sure, we can work on that now. Tell me when you feel anxious.

N: If I'm lying down. It comes to me when I'm by myself and not talking to someone. It comes to me when I'm not stimulated by another person. I tend to fixate—that's exactly what happens—I fixate on, "Oh, am I going to be able to swallow?" It's swallowing. I think it's probably something that most of the time, we don't think about doing, right? Autonomic or something. The minute I stop and start looking at swallowing and waiting for it to happen, it stops happening. It feeds itself—the fear.

RM: This lack of swallowing—that triggers your fear?

N: Yes. I want to swallow, and I cannot swallow. Maybe I'm not ready to swallow—we don't swallow every second—but now it's become such a different feel.

RM: This started with the dry throat?

N: The panic started yesterday evening. Anna was here; we were talking, and I truly could not swallow. It really was an emergency. She was quick, got me upright, and got some water down me, and then I was OK. Then it just started snowballing. The dryness was so severe that I could not swallow, even when I really had to. But as soon we got the humidifier on, it got better physically. It's just not psychologically better.

RM: Your confidence has been shaken. This experience taps into what you talked about last week, about being frightened. This is a variation of the fear that you felt. You've taken one giant step to solving this by getting a humidifier. You have been traumatized, and there is residual anxiety.

N: That's exactly what it is!

Commentary: This episode illustrates the connection between disturbing physical symptoms and intrusive thoughts. Nell's difficulty swallowing triggers fear and panic, which, in turn, foster the intrusive thought, "I won't be able to swallow," when she has a dry mouth. This thought sets in motion muscle tension and anxiety, which exacerbate the symptom of difficulty swallowing and suffocation. It is a downward spiral.

The difficulty swallowing and the accompanying fear can be reduced. A method for coping is to either lose, lessen, or live with the symptom or problem. This simple "three L's" way to think about a complex situation can be reassuring, allowing the patient to conceive the possibility of living with a lessened symptom or modified problem. In

Nell's situation, she is losing her swallowing problem and lessening her fear.

For now, Nell is very responsive to a breathing intervention and reassurance that she can manage her swallowing problem and fear. We have done deep-breathing and guided-imagery exercises in prior sessions. While I believe that she can lessen or perhaps even lose her fear, I am acutely aware that symptoms can spiral out of control at the end. I wonder if my reassurance rings hollow, not so much to her, but to me. Can I really protect her from this terrible possibility at the end? Even with preparation, death always seems to come too fast and with surprises. I hope to be by her side if she needs help at the end and must prepare her to leave this world without me.

RM: Let's do some deep breathing now. (Here, I direct her in a 10-minute, deep-breathing exercise.)

RM: How was that?

N: Good. I could not swallow, though. See, I did swallow then. That's what I need to get hold of. I can swallow, except maybe I am not ready that minute.

RM: You just swallowed. It was a surprise?

N: Because I tried a moment before to swallow, and nothing happened. Maybe swallowing is not something I can command, and I tried to command it. I'm trying to let myself swallow, so I'll know when I can. I'm pushing the system.

RM: Hmm, well, you're making me want to swallow now, too.

N: (Laughs.) I'm sorry.

RM: I'm paying attention to swallowing.

N: You'll start getting crazy like me! (Laughs.)

RM: No, you are not that crazy (laughs), but you are stuck in your head on swallowing. Now, if you drink water, you can swallow; you can do that. So have you considered, if you're stuck, take a sip?

N: That is what I do. I have to sit up, sit up and get something in there to swallow, and then the system works.

RM: Then you are good?

N: Yes, what's funny is this. It's like burping a baby. There is usually some air down there.

RM: Sure, you're getting some up pressure, some air? Your body is telling you things, "I'm not ready to swallow" or "You are different now," and the way to manage that is the way that you just did—lessening or losing the symptom by putting your problem-solving skills to work and relaxing as best you can by taking a deep breath. Let's talk about the scary part. Tell me about your fear, being scared.

N: I know it's chutzpah on my part to dictate to fate, which obviously has not been listening to me anyway. I really do not want to suffocate. That's scary. The swallowing and struggling for air are scary.

RM: There is no reason to suffocate. Your lungs are not filling up with fluid. They are not filling up with tumor, which would create that sense of suffocation, so that is not on the horizon. Periodically, you might struggle for air. I will talk to Dr. T about it. We are taking steps to reduce the symptoms of suffocation. Tumor growth is causing this indirectly through pressure on your diaphragm. It is scary, and you are learning to master your fear.

N: Yes, right.

RM: I think you have told me it's your liver that will fail, and that will cause your body to start shutting down?

N: That's what Dr. T said.

RM: He tells me, too. I will ask him again about this sensation. Today, he said that if you got in pain and distress, the morphine is the route to help settle yourself.

N: I really leaned on it yesterday and today because it not only reduces the pain but also relaxes those muscles.

RM: Relaxes you and then you can breathe more easily. Tension and anxiety can make breathing harder. Those momentary feelings of panic you have when you're lying down or when you're getting tired will subside with deep breathing and with the knowledge that you are not suffocating. It's a temporary struggle; you will come out of it with water, breathing, sitting up. Your body is undergoing tremendous change. One way to manage your thoughts is deep breathing, which you are doing. It's almost like Lamaze breathing.

N: Which I was never present for. Were you?

RM: I was taught when my wife and I went through Lamaze training, but I was not the one delivering!

N: Yes, a big difference!

Commentary: *Sometimes, information is all Nell needs to understand the changes in her body and to manage her symptoms. Being aware of what is happening can be a powerful source of reassurance as the body goes through such radical changes, as this dialogue illustrates.*

RM: We are talking about a simple technique—attending to natural breathing and a deep cleansing breath. If you get in a place where you feel this difficulty swallowing and panic arising, use your technique for breathing and problem-solving—drinking a sip of water—to lessen the symptom and master fear. You can also let it be and accept that you are not swallowing—just let it be. So now, just lean back and close your eyes, breathe in and out, just in and out slowly and naturally. (Nell practices directed breathing for several minutes.) That's right.

N: That short exercise helped. Sometimes just sitting up will do it. That's good to know. So tell me again—what Dr. T was saying was that this organ shutdown is the route to expect. He characterized it as just sleeping more and more and more.

RM: Yes, and not choking.

N: See, it's all tumor here around my stomach. All the way around to the spine now. It is so big, it starts here and goes around my entire abdomen.

RM: Does it hurt?

N: It is hurting more. It hurts a lot. My two 15-milligram morphine tablets don't quite cover the four hours. If it keeps being
that way, we probably need to increase the fentanyl patch.

RM: If you need to transition to a different dose of fentanyl, talk to
your nurse or Dr. T. You can call me, too. Dr. T and his team
are knowledgeable about pain management. If you run into
a snag like the oxygen humidifier, I can act as your advocate.
You have enough to do without chasing the medical team
around for medication.

N: It was crazy. It was truly crazy.

RM: You're doing your part, managing the changes in your body.
A source of worry now is the possibility of suffocating. That
does not have to happen and won't happen, all right?

N: Say it again, please.

RM: That should not happen. We are getting your team in place to
make sure you have good movement now, good preparation,
to make the leap on your own time.

*Commentary: I am aware that my reassurance has limitations even
as I say these words. Nobody can guarantee how death might arrive,
yet I'm hopeful that with the good care provided by hospice, close
surveillance by Dr. T, and regular contact with me, Nell can avoid
the panic of suffocation and have a death of her choosing. Nobody
controls death. At best we can guide it, prepare, and respond as best
we can.*

N: I am the least in-charge person. Do you think it can be on my
own terms? I feel like I'm skating in the dark.

RM: Skating in the dark?

N: Can you imagine that feeling? Ice skating in the dark?

RM: Yes, and that is a scary feeling.

N: That is scary. I do not want to dwell on that. I'm sorry. I'm a
coward.

RM: You are no coward. Here, take my hand and hold on as you skate in the dark. You will come out. (Long pause.) You can skate to the light.

Commentary: As I hold Nell's hand, I am aware of the times I have seen two people tethered together, one blind, trusting, the other with sight, leading, guiding. I hope I can be Nell's guide now, holding her hand as she makes her way, as she finds safe passage through Cancerland. The image of ice skating in the dark and the fear that might accompany it are powerful. I hope my presence can ease Nell's fear.

N: I have to trust.

RM: Yes, trust your body, your spirit, and your caregivers to know how to make this move. You are doing well—juggling tasks, being in charge, orchestrating with the medical team.

N: They don't know they're a team! (Laughs.) It is very interesting, isn't it?

RM: Yes, it is. That is part of the problem—how the team works or does not at times. I have a poem that might help. It's called "Are You Afraid" by Mary Oliver.[1] Would you like to hear it?

N: I would.

RM: This comes out of our conversation last week, when you spoke of feeling afraid. That was the first time I recognized how powerful the fear had become, how strong it was. Oliver's poem speaks of fear (see Box 5.1).

N: That is a spectacular poem! I was listening hard!

RM: Mary Oliver is a special poet. Her words speak to fear, letting go. Part of this is letting go, letting be, but also knowing when to reach for the glass of water.

Commentary: The word inspiration, *often linked to poetry, comes from the Latin* inspiratus, *the past participle of* inspirare, *to breathe into. Nell needs inspiration now as she fears suffocation. The Oliver poem (Box 5.1) expresses two themes, fear and forever (eternity),*

Box 5.1 Are You Afraid?

Mary Oliver

Are you afraid?
    The ear of corn knows whereof it is plucked

Are you afraid?
    The wind moves this way and that way, something
        is pushing it.

Are you afraid?
    Somewhere a thousand swans are flying
        through the winter's worst storm.

They are white and shining, their black beaks
    open a little, the red tongues flash.

Now and *now* and *now* and *now* their heavy wings
    rise and fall as they move across the sky.
Goodbye to the gold finches
in their silver baskets.
Goodbye to the pilot whales, and the curl of their spines
in the crisp waves.
Goodbye to the grasshopper.
Goodbye to the pond lilies, the turtle with her
cat's head.
Goodbye to the lion's mane floating in the harbor
like a spangled vale.

Goodbye to the moon uprising in the east.
Goodbye to the going forth, and coming home

Goodbye to the going forth and holding on and worrying.
Goodbye to the engine of breath.

The knee sings its anguish
The ears fill with the sound of ringing water.
The muscles of the eyes pull towards sleep.

Goodbye to the swaying trees.
Goodbye to the black triangles of the winter sea.
Goodbye to the oranges, the prick of their fragrance.
Goodbye to the fox and sparrow,
goodbye to the blue winged teal.
Goodbye to lettuce, and the pale turnip,
and the gatherings of the rice fields.
Goodbye to the morning light.
Goodbye to the gold finches
    and their wavering songs.
Slowly
up the hill,
like a thicket of white flowers,
forever
is coming.

that Nell has discussed over the course of our work together. The prospect of some form of existence after our earthly life comforts her yet does not conform to the common notion of a triple-decker universe of heaven, earth, and hell. Believing she will somehow rejoin the great circle of life is helpful to her. The poem's ending, "forever / is coming," helps to make her suffering bearable. Contemplating that forever is coming is both comforting and mind-blowing. I am headed to forever, too. Where are we going? Where did we come from?

N: I was so looking forward to talking with you about this because I know that you are familiar with the physiological level
as well as the psychological level. You would not tell me a story.
(Laughs.)

RM: No, I would not. I believe in you.

N: I am glad to have your reassurance because, in a sense, this is
not manageable, but maybe it is manageable?

RM: The physical sensations are uncomfortable, and you can
manage them. You are managing them well, although there
are times when you feel scared—"I can't get my breath." Your
breath will always come back to you, Nell, even when it feels
lost. Part of it is letting go.

N: That is a paradox.

RM: Letting go of your breath to let it come back—yes, it is a paradox. You've had a busy week, it seems, and you did the work
of getting your breath back. The spirit is back, too.

N: That is a good way to put it.

RM: How are you feeling right now?

N: Just a little uncomfortable. I cannot take another morphine.
I lost track of when I took it—I think about 5 o'clock—so I'm
only halfway through my four hours.

RM: You are noticing the pain now; it's poking through. On a zero-
to-10 scale, where are you with the pain right now?

N: Eight.

RM: That is too high.

N: I agree. That's not my favorite range. I could call it seven.

RM: You could call it seven? But it hurts! This is the time to decide if you want to do something about it—to call and talk
to your hospice nurse. You are only halfway through to your
next dose. It's not good to spend two hours in the seven and
eight pain range. You may be making a transition to needing a
higher dose of medication.

N: I think yes, I am. I think I will wait until tomorrow and call the
clinic instead and start at Dr. T's end with this. Only because

Audrey, as sweet as she is, has not proven herself as a person to get results.

RM: Audrey is your hospice nurse?

N: Yes, she is very sweet. She is the one who called at 8 a.m. to see whether the humidifier had arrived. I think I'll just call Dr. T and leave word that we need to talk about my pain.

Commentary: Nell frequently refers to her highly valued and respected medical oncologist, Dr. T. I am fortunate to be on the faculty with him in the same section of Hematology and Oncology. We attend meetings together and often talk because our offices are in the same area. This puts me in a unique position to be useful to Nell, helping her to navigate the situation. Physicians don't usually agree to manage pain medication after their patients are referred to home hospice care, and Dr. T's continued supervision is a great benefit to Nell since he knows her. She trusts him to always act in her best interest.

RM: Your current dosage is the patch plus the pills for breakthrough pain.

N: I can cheat by an hour or so, I know—that's what the CNAs tell me.

RM: All right. I would not call it cheating; I would say adapting, being flexible to the situation.

N: Especially when you know that when your next four hours show up, you'll be asleep. (Laughs.) So maybe in an hour, I will take another one. I am getting sleepy now. Thank you.

RM: Can I get you anything?

N: I wish you were here all the time. You are so reassuring.

RM: I am here now. I am with you.

Commentary: Nell's wish tugs at my heart and speaks to her strong need for a companion who can negotiate the rough emotional waters that often accompany the end times. Al's presence, while comforting, cannot provide all that Nell needs. I am glad I can be with her in these moments, and I hope my reassurance is not hollow in the end—eight weeks from now.

N: When you put your hand on my tumor, it was wonderful. Could you put your hand back? Your hand is warm, very warm. Did you do Reiki?

RM: I had a person say to me once that I had healing hands, but I have not been trained in Reiki.

Commentary: Psychologists' code of ethics provide guidelines for touching patients. I have no hesitation about responding to Nell's request, even though my profession might see it as close to a boundary violation. These rules are designed to protect therapists and patients from sexual contact, not the healing touch exerted in this situation. I can help Nell manage her pain and the parasitic cancer she feels bulging from her center by placing my hand on her liver, gorged with tumor.

N: You *do* have a healing touch.

RM: Thank you. I am wishing you healing through me, your good spirit, and the wisdom of your body. Your body is not acting exactly the way you want it, but it's acting the best it can with an uninvited tumor on board. What did you call it—alien?

N: Probably. It is certainly a parasite. I love what Belleruth Naparstek says on the CD you gave me—that we are born knowing how to die.[2] It's hardwired in every child. We just lose sight of it as we go along in life. It is mystifying—born knowing how to die. It's part of our organism, in every organic thing—we know all we need to know.

RM: And that knowledge is coming to you now, here, in your head and heart.

N: The knowledge is almost unrecognizable. It comes disguised as fear.

RM: Fear comes to visit, and you can smile at the same time. You have a way of meeting fear, acknowledging and accepting it. You watch movies or basketball to take your mind away from fear or pain. Maybe you have something scheduled for tonight?

Commentary: Distraction is a useful technique to minimize intrusive thoughts and the experience of pain. It has proven effective for a number of physical and mental health conditions. We tell people who are angry to count to 10 or to remove themselves from the situation before doing something rash. Research has found that distraction can reduce the number of pain signals that reach the brain by triggering the release of endogenous opioids in the body.[3]

N: (Laughs.) We haven't discussed it yet. I would like to finish the *Sopranos* tape that we have, but Al is so sweet to watch TV with me. He's started to get addicted to it, too. I don't want to impose *The Sopranos* on him. Maybe we will watch *Foyle's War*.

RM: OK, I'll take my leave now. See you next time.

N: Thank you.

Final Commentary: I try to end our conversations on an upbeat note of hope. As I leave tonight, I recognize that Nell is mastering her fear. I wonder if we should attempt to go deeper into her fear rather than "managing" it away. The intensity of death talk can be overwhelming. I look for cues from Nell about how far she wants to go into her own fear. We have just made a connection to the fear that stalks her; now, as I leave, she chuckles and looks forward to time with Al and the distraction of their evening television programs. Have I helped her avoid a more useful encounter with death or gone just far enough? Am I avoiding the inevitability of mortality? These are the questions to ponder before our next conversation, where Nell will speak of new insights about meeting, accepting, and yielding to death.

Notes

1. Oliver, M. (2000). *The leaf and the cloud* (p. 40). Boston: Da Capo Press.
2. Naparstek, B. Accepting death. https://healingjourneys.org/
3. Sprenger, C., Eippert, F., Finsterbusch, J., Bingel, U., Rose, M., & Büchel, C. (2012). Attention modulates spinal cord responses to pain. *Current Biology, 22*(11), 1019–1022.

6

April 27, 2005—Holding On

". . . the present is understood as precariously binding the past and future together: the moment we try to pin it down, it is either 'no more' or "not yet."
>   Arendt, H. (1978). *The life of the mind. Two: Willing.*
>   (p. 13). New York: Harcourt, Inc.

Main Themes: Facing, accepting, and yielding to death.

Meaning-making and managing physical decline in mortal time are recurrent themes in our conversations. Nell succinctly describes her plan for making sense of death: Face it, accept it, and yield to it. However, she recognizes that this simple prescription is not easy to fulfill. Part of facing death requires detaching from activities that give meaning and link her to the broader world. On most days now, she lacks the energy to engage the outside world; she is housebound.

In his autobiography, Paul Kalanithi presents an example of yielding as he describes his slow decline due to lung cancer.[1] Like Nell, he faced his illness directly, with grace, until the very end, literally writing from his deathbed. When he wrote all he could, his wife stepped in to add a final dimension to the book. She addresses the question Nell grapples with throughout these dialogues: What makes life worth living when death is imminent?

This session begins with a discussion of security objects and Nell telling me about Fr. Jay, her parish priest, anointing her and giving her a ceramic angel. She finds comfort in consoling iconography and holding on to her rosary, a crucifix, angels, the Buddha.

Dialogue 6

N: Here, what do you think of this little angel?

RM: I like it. It's very nice.

N: Fr. Jay gave it to me and suggested that I have a cross here, too. I do have a cross in the other room. He said to have something I can get hold of when I'm anxious. I also have a rosary someone brought for me.

RM: And now you have an angel. It is important to have a meaningful physical object to hold. And it can be helpful to hold the hands of those who love you as well as the voice and spirit of those who you want to keep with you always. What is most important for the journey is already inside you—in your head and heart.

N: Yes, it helps. Can you hold my hand?

RM: Yes, I can. Especially in the night, someone or some item to hold if you are afraid. If you awake in the night, then you can put the angel or rosary in your hand.

Commentary: Holding Nell's hand feels true, like an act of kindness. I believe kindness is the most important gift we can leave in this world. It remains in the hearts, minds, and souls of those we touch. Everything else turns to dust. How will we be remembered after we are gone? "She was kind." Kindness, only kindness, lasts.

N: Once . . . you started to talk about this idea of holding something, but I do not remember what it was.

RM: You were talking about feeling less engaged with the *New York Times* and different things, and we spoke of letting go of some things and holding others.

N: Yes, I've always really, really appreciated things like National Public Radio in particular and the *New York Times* as indications of my engagement in the world, of our being one human community, in an active real way.

RM: Yes, sure.

N: And most often expressed politically, I think, in the affirmation that we are all in this together, in the human experience. My friend Anna in particular has been very good about bringing the *Times* since I am not getting out anywhere to get it. Lately, Anna has fallen off from that. It is interesting because, at the same time, my sense of urgency about having a newspaper connection to the human community—that sense of urgency is diminishing. I know I am connected to the human community. I do not have to get the *New York Times* every day to remind me. (Laughs.)

RM: You are changing, making adjustments, becoming connected to a different reality.

N: It's not only that I have lost interest; it's that I don't have the magnitude of spirit to engage both this dying process and being a politically engaged human being. The process of dying is taking all of my psychic energy. When someone brings the *Times*, I find myself not reading pieces that I read in the past. That's it, for what it's worth.

RM: You're not as connected to National Public Radio or to the *New York Times* or reading partly because you are deeply engaged with the process of dying, with letting go to a new world.

N: Yes. What I did not realize is how much work it is. It really is hard work! Every once in a while, I remind myself it takes character to face what's going on and accept it. These are the steps: Face it, accept it, and then yield to it. That number three is the hardest because that is where the trust is absolute. Absolute trust is absolutely required to do step three—yielding.

RM: Yielding—and you are yielding now?

N: I'm working on it. It is not something that comes naturally or automatically. It is, at some level, a matter of character to accept what is going on. It is an act of will. It is going to be forced upon me anyway. I can go resisting (laughs), or I can go willingly. I am slowly getting to willingly. It's that thing that Jesus got to, to use a local example. I do not know how the Buddha felt when he was dying (laughs).

Commentary: Nell has accepted her fate and inevitable death; she has spoken openly about her fears for many weeks. She has been imagining what death might be like and hoping to engineer a good ending while actively attending to practical matters. She is also learning how to transcend her fear by managing her physical symptoms with medicine and psychological techniques. Her full grieving has not yet emerged. Perhaps by yielding she means experiencing the grief of her mortality and death.

RM: Pretty good examples—Jesus and the Buddha, too. You have always been open to the life you have, your breast cancer diagnosis, and what it means. At the beginning of our talks, you told me your doctors said this was not curable. You had accepted that fact. Now you are entering a new stage of labor, moving out of this world and into the new world. It is laborious.

N: Lots of work!

RM: And there are times when you feel frightened, although right now you look very peaceful.

N: Fr. Jay anointing me with oil really helped.[2] It was wonderful. It all went so quickly, I can't put my finger on what he did and said that was so wonderful, but he was present, and he seemed to understand that I was frightened—that you should be— that it's natural to be frightened. He was just very strong. I am leaning hard these days. I am leaning on you! I am leaning on the faith (laughs), and I am leaning on Al.

RM: Yes, I see. It's good to lean, to trust, and to know that Al is right here with you. I will leave my voice with you. In the middle of the night, you can call it forth. We will do a little bit of work on that before we stop tonight, so you will have another method at night in addition to your mental strategies, your spirit, the rosary, and the little angel to hold. You are managing what is in your heart and head, what it all means. You are working hard and well.

N: Yes, thank you. Do you have any questions for me?

RM: About life, about death? About how you're doing?

N: All of the above.

RM: I wonder with you about facing, accepting, and yielding to death. You are showing me a path of bravery and wonder at dying. Your spirit is willing; your body is changing. I wonder with you and travel with you and Al as far as I can go. Your friends are with you, and you are traveling well. However, even in good travels, there are storms, wind, lack of a humidifier for the oxygen, and unanswered phone calls to hospice.

N: (Chuckles.) Truly!

RM: So those are some of my thoughts. And what of your questions?

N: I think I've asked you all of my questions. I was glad I called you last night. I felt stupid. I should have done it earlier in the day, but I did not. I didn't know how (laugh), so I didn't want to do it.

RM: You didn't know how?

N: I mean, I knew how mechanically to call you on the phone, but I wasn't exactly sure what I was calling for, which is probably the main reason I should have called.

RM: That's right. (Both laugh.) I am with you.

N: It was very, very helpful. I was scared. I am grateful to you for talking to me yesterday.

Commentary: Nell called after 5 p.m. A phone call is a simple way to reach out, yet Nell hesitated. She is very independent and accustomed to handling her own problems; she did not want to place demands on me. The therapy process produces intense feelings of dependence on the therapist that can be uncomfortable for both patient and therapist. In order to manage such intense feelings, all therapists establish physical and emotional boundaries. For some patients, I provide my cell phone number and am accessible through email and our institutional medical record portal 24/7, although I may not be able to reply immediately. I respond to an identified emergency or note of urgency as quickly as possible. Since Nell is contending with her final days, I do my best to be available to her. I received her recorded message after 5 p.m. and called her that night. I'm glad I can be useful and hope to help her manage the fear near the end. I welcomed her call.

RM: I am traveling with you. There are times like yesterday when we can use the phone to make sense out of a very scary experience that threw you off stride. You were off stride only for a short time. It still reverberates—there are echoes and aftershocks—and yet you have come back to yourself.

N: It's because of your steadiness. The network of care is holding. It's not perfect, but it is holding. It could be perfect, and it will be perfect, if ever the medical people get it together, if they ever integrate the clinical/medical side and the hospice side. Then everybody would be in the same building and able to talk face to face—that would be very beautiful. As we are, I think of it like the highways in California after the mudslides this winter—the highways with surfaces all broken up, and the pieces do not connect with one another. There is a big drop-off to the next step in communication, like getting hold of my hospice nurse Audrey and so forth, getting everybody talking about the same thing. And of course, me not knowing what it is that everyone's talking about! (Laughs.)

RM: We're talking about safe passage for you and the necessary steps to help that happen, including good communication.

Then there is the very specific mechanics of working toward comfort, no suffocation for sure, peacefulness for you.

N: Oh, yes, please.

RM: That's the path we are on with your team. We know that there are snags within the network. You are wise to have backup, and you have Al here, Anna, and Audrey of hospice.

N: I think that is where I wish the highway were one piece because I do not know Audrey well enough.

RM: You don't know her well enough, and you're not sure about her?

N: Not sure about her ability or experience. She wants to be reassuring, and sometimes her desire to be reassuring can overtake everything else. I'm not sure about the quality of the information or advice I get.

RM: OK, tell me more about it.

N: She is very, very sweet, but she has not been down this road [and is not] planning to be in the near future. . . . She cannot know exactly what might happen to me. She is humble in that way, which is good. If she were coming in and being apodictic, it would not make sense. I miss the impression of professionalism that the clinic gives. The professionalism gives me confidence in what they're doing. That's not there with the informal encounters.

RM: The professionalism helps you feel they know what to do. If a problem comes up, you want a technical expert. If you are in pain, you want to knock that out. If you feel like suffocating, you want that to stop. You want experienced guidance.

N: Yes!

RM: Professionalism from your caregivers is a reasonable expectation. Those are the same hopes I have for you. If you are suffocating, we need to stop that; if you are in pain, we need to stop that with methods that work. You are working well. You're using the pain medicine, and you've gotten the oxygen situation straightened out. Those are good steps.

N: (Emphatic) Yes! The increase in the pain patch is very good; I am not getting much pain, yet there is one area that the pain medication doesn't hold, but I'm not writhing much. Right here— feel this tumor.

RM: Yes, does it hurt now?

N: It doesn't hurt. I took a pill at 5:45. But at times the pain comes on suddenly. It's the part that goes first, and it's right here— sort of the root. (Nell points and places my hand on her side.) The root of all evil is right here (laughs).

Commentary: Contemplating meaning when the body is in pain is difficult, if not impossible. Nell is an excellent communicator, which helps her team know exactly where her pain is and when it strikes. Pain management is both an art and a science, and good communication is crucial to success. I feel responsible for helping Nell to navigate through her episodes of pain to reach satisfactory management. Pain can make sustained conversation impossible.

RM: This is where the pain is? It starts here? If you get the medicine at the right time, it will hold for a couple of hours?

N: Yes. Dr. T has changed it so that I can take the morphine as often as every 2 hours. Audrey is putting in a call about oxygen. He apparently had prescribed a level two of the oxygen for me. Fortunately, the guy off the street—the guy who came to install the oxygen tank—told me it was set at two, but "you can do whatever you want with it" (laughs).

RM: Really?

N: I asked him, "What level is it?" and he said, "Two." I guess I looked like "Oh, that's not very first class" (laughs), and he replied that I could adjust it, so I adjusted it—first, to two-and-a-half for quite a while and then three and then just a little more. Today, Audrey showed Sally how to refill the water bottle so that Sally will take some responsibility for keeping that up.

RM: And your oxygen is adjustable up as high as—?

N: Yes, I think up to six. Sally thought I was to stop at five. There is some kind of reaction that sets in if you're pushing it too hard. She is going to ask Dr. T to give us a range between two and five.

RM: Great. You are managing this well. Before this oxygen arrived, you were feeling very low.

N: Punk, and naturally I did not understand that. Now I do.

RM: Yes, really, punk. Your body needs oxygen for energy. Did you have labs drawn today?

N: No, that's only once a month. They have to flush the port-a-cath once a month to avoid infection, and I guess that's when they will do labs, so it's just once a month since we quit chemo.

RM: Is there anything else on your mind now? If not, we will shift to practice the technique of settling yourself.

N: I would like you to do that. I would like to just preserve your voice.

Commentary: We stopped taping for 15 minutes to do a relaxation imagery session and to briefly discuss it. The guided-imagery sessions I conducted with Nell were facilitated by peaceful music and specific instructions. I'd start by asking her to pay attention to her breathing, the music, and my voice. I would ask her to relax and to let go of intrusive thoughts or sounds. She would then take three deep, cleansing breaths and try to imagine a safe place—to see that place in her mind's eye. The safe-place image can be very comforting. After about ten minutes of peaceful breathing and guided imagery, I gently ask her to return to full awareness of her surroundings yet remain fully relaxed.[3]

N: I wish you had recorded what you just said. That was very beautiful and healing. If you haven't recorded it, you should, as part of whatever you are putting together. It was very, very profound.

RM: Thank you. You did record it in your memory.

N: Well, I want other people to have it, too. (Laughs.) I can't remember yesterday anymore. There were many people yesterday.

RM: Yesterday is a blur. You have little sense of yesterday? Your memory is more attuned to a sense of movement, and that's enough—that's fine. You're noticing a shift in the days, which is good.

N: It was funny—Sally was here. Sally heard me making noise when I was trying to wake up from my dream, and she came into my room. I told her about the dream. Before she left, she came in and took my hands and reminded me about trust, which we talked about before. She didn't pray—sometimes she bursts into prayer—she didn't do that, but we made an intense connection. It was very, very nice, and I thought about last night, when I was surrendering to facing the necessity of sleeping, I thought about it, and I held on to that, held on to talking with you on the phone and just prayed for strength, for character, to let myself go into sleep and to wake up.

RM: You have strong character, but even someone like you with strong character can be afraid. You went through the fear yesterday and mastered it. You will continue to do that should you encounter fear again. You have guardians to help you; you have medicines to help, a whole menu, to help with this trip. Now, tonight you may fall into a deep sleep. You are tuckered out. Can I get you anything before I leave?

N: I don't think so. I'll watch *The Sopranos* with Al when you leave.

RM: OK. I have another poem by Mary Oliver. It's called "Poppies."[4]

N: Yes, please (Box 6.1).

N: That is wonderful. Beautiful . . .

RM: Take care until next time.

Final Commentary: Nell takes comfort in poetry, especially the poems of Mary Oliver. She closes her eyes and listens carefully. Sometimes, she dozes lightly, always coming alert when I stop speaking. Oliver's poems are soothing, yet contain the invitation to understand that loss is always with us, even when the flowers bloom. In "Poppies" (Box 6.1), the flower "shines like a miracle" but "Of course nothing stops the cold." This poem resonates with themes of loss and promise. Nell is comforted by the imagery in poetry, highlighting

Box 6.1   Poppies

Mary Oliver

The poppies send up their
orange flares; swaying
in the wind, their congregations
are a levitation

of bright dust, of thin
and lacy leaves.
There isn't a place
in this world that doesn't

sooner or later drown
in the indigos of darkness,
but now, for a while,
the roughage

shines like a miracle
as it floats above everything
with its yellow hair.
Of course nothing stops the cold,

black, curved blade
from hooking forward—
of course
loss is the great lesson.

But I also say this: that light
is an invitation
to happiness,
and that happiness,

when it's done right,
is a kind of holiness,
palpable and redemptive.
Inside the bright fields,

touched by their rough and spongy gold,
I am washed and washed
in the river
of earthly delight—

and what are you going to do—
what can you do
about it—
deep, blue night?

the beauty of nature and the connection between all things. She believes in the power of connection and community. In our next conversation she reveals an epiphany of contentment and "feeling free to go or stay now."

Notes

1. Kalanithi, P. (2016). *When breath becomes air*. New York: Random House.
2. Anointing of the Sick is a sacrament of the Catholic Church and recognized as a rite by the Lutheran, Anglican, and Methodist churches. Some Anglicans also hold it as a sacrament. It is one of the three sacraments that make up the last rites, which we discussed in Chapter 3.
3. This type of meditative exercise is illustrated in Levine, S. (1987). *Healing into life and death*. New York: Anchor Books.
4. Oliver, M. (1992). *New and selected poems*. Boston: Beacon Press.

7

May 3, 2005—An Epiphany

To sleep! perchance to dream: – ay, there's
    the rub;
For in that sleep of death what dreams may
    Come

Shakespeare, *Hamlet*, Act 3, Scene 1, ll. 65–67

Main Themes: An egregious boundary violation by a professional caregiver, an epiphany about death, reassurance from a chaplain, and managing symptoms.

In this dialogue, Nell describes a very disruptive visit from Kristin, a private-duty nurse caregiver I had enlisted, and a helpful visit from the hospice chaplain, who tells her of God's promise: You will not be alone at the end. It greatly comforts her. Being homebound has increased her sense of isolation and fear that she will die alone.

I emphasize how well she is managing the physical obstacles to dying. The tasks of daily living now take much of her time. I want to be useful to her and regularly question her about how she is doing. I have accompanied others on this road and have seen bad deaths unfold as the body deteriorates. I want to help Nell avoid a painful death.

She begins our conversation by describing the relief she experiences at night in dreams where she is not moored to her bed. I am delighted to hear it and to learn that our meetings are a welcome distraction from the slow deterioration of her body and episodes of fear. I'm pleased that even when the topic is mortality, our conversations can be healing and surprised she describes them as fun.

Dialogue 7

N: I woke up this morning wondering why I sleep so well. I sleep beautifully, even when I sleep with my mouth open, which you are not supposed to do (laughs)—I should be drinking the oxygen through my nose and all of that. I woke up and realized that I slept very comfortably, whereas during the day I experience a lot more discomfort. During the day, the disease process is always in the back of my mind. When I'm sleeping, it's not. I'm having these wonderful dreams where I go places, do delicious things, and have adventures.

RM: That's wonderful!

N: It is fun. This recording project of ours takes my mind off monitoring how I'm feeling, yet thinking about dying is irresistible in one sense.

RM: Tell me more about that.

N: At some level, I can't *not* be thinking about death all the time, but it's debilitating. So this conversation we're having is actually fun. It takes my mind off death.

RM: That's nice! Talking about your life and reading the transcript of our conversation puts you in a different frame so that you are not thinking about death all the time? Yet going through these transcripts must set you to ruminating.

N: That's where it's helpful to have the editorial liberty to say a little more. Here, when we're talking, maybe we stumble around sometimes (laughs), yet there is synergy here and learning.

RM: Absolutely, synergy. You said to me once, "Well, I don't think I have enough energy to do editing." Has that changed?

N: You did throw me a challenge! (Laughs.) I am doing it. It was fun today. I didn't wake up until noon, so I didn't spend the whole day working on editing, naturally, but that's to be expected.

RM: Tell me what you're learning and discovering.

N: Not enough material yet. I haven't discovered anything yet. However, I'm aware of not going so quickly. I just read our first interview. I can see from the middle of February until now, there has been quite a lot of change in my perception. It will be interesting to see that play itself out as we go through this series of interviews.

RM: You can see the change in you?

N: I have changed. The things that preoccupied, concerned, or frightened me when we first talked on tape have changed to other things now. (Pause.) I'm trying to get my mind back into the present. I'm trying to remember where we are in our conversation now, and I'm not succeeding.

RM: Can you let it be? You're distracted now; your attention will come back. I see the *New York Times* open on your bed though, so that has changed. (Laughs.)

N: It's baaaccckkk! (Laughs.) Al just brought the *Times* home today. This is his day on campus, so he brought it with him, and I was charmed. (Laughs.)

Commentary: *For the first time in our dialogues, Nell loses track of her thoughts. This loss of focus can happen for a variety of reasons, including physical symptoms and pain medication. Fortunately, it does not preoccupy her for long. Patients can become very distressed at the first sign of mental status changes, wondering if they are a sign of cancer progression. Nell needs only a moment to recover her sense of humor, imitating a variation on the phrase "I'm back," which appears in several movies. She will speak more about her changing perception today and in subsequent meetings.*

RM: Have you been reading the *Times*?

N: Yes, some. There is a kind of movement back and forth on different things like reading. I do not want to be alone, and reading helps. Al goes to campus on Tuesdays. Sally only stays until 2 o'clock at the latest, and he gets home closer to 4. I just asked her to stay the extra couple of hours.

RM: Yes, good.

N: There is something bottomless about the thought of being alone here.

RM: Bottomless—that sounds lonely. I think it's good for you to have somebody here. You're not quite as agile as you could be. I talked to Kristin today about being with you.

Commentary: I could have taken this opportunity to expand on Nell's feeling of loneliness, which can accelerate for isolated, homebound cancer patients, but quickly moved to practical considerations about having someone present. I try to follow the general principle of "empathy before information-giving/problem-solving," as patients want to be heard above all else. In this case, solving the problem could have come later after expanding on the feeling of "something bottomless." My alacrity at assuring her someone could be present overshadowed her feelings.

N: Yes, talk to me about Kristin.

RM: I want to talk to you about her as I know she came over on Saturday for a rushed visit. I was asking her about additional care—people to look after you—and she said it might be time to consider a nurse to come in. That is the main thing that I wanted to talk with you about, given how you feel. I talked to Audrey as well. She called yesterday morning.

N: OK.

RM: She is working with you to assure you will be protected from the feeling of suffocation. I talked with her about how important that is. I asked, "Can you help Nell avoid the feeling of suffocation?" She answered, "Yes."

N: Did she have a strategy for that—for what we can do? Is there some strategy?

RM: The strategy is twofold. One: As your body, mind, and spirit let go, you may be less cognizant of bodily sensations. Two: The use of medication for sedation to make sure that you do not have a sense of suffocation. Those are the two strategies. One is natural—what your body does—and the other is having a nurse available to provide medication as needed, potentially in the middle of the night if you wake up. That is something to consider.

N: Staffing up?

RM: Yes, essentially. I'm saying that based on what Kristin said. She has hospice experience.

N: I want to tell you about Kristin. She did two very big no-nos on Saturday. First off, she calls on Friday. She calls *me*, mind you! She calls me, and she wants to come see me, and so reluctantly, I said, "Well, it would need to be very short, but how is 2:00 on Saturday?" You know, my dear friend Pat Toole was leaving for California, and she was coming Saturday, too.

RM: Pat called me and told me what happened.

N: I know. That's how I know you know Pat is going to California. Pat was scheduled to come at 2:30. We had the most wonderful visit. It was 3 o'clock, and we were discussing the sacrament of confession and how amazingly powerful I had found it. She's Presbyterian. She was just telling me how they do it in her church, and I'm really having an intimate conversation. Kristin arrives at the door at 3 o'clock, not 2 o'clock. Al meets her and says Nell is with someone. Kristin says, "Oh, I won't be very long," and she just barges right in and comes into the bedroom—not "Am I interrupting you?" or "Could I leave and come back?"—she barges right into the bedroom and wants to start talking, and Pat, being the polite person, unlike Kristin, gets up to go, and I said, "Pat, please do not leave this room."

RM: Very intrusive.

N: And Kristin said, "Well, I just need a hug." I thought, "It's all about what you need—that's what it is." So I gave her a damn hug! She is here, and she starts tickling my feet. My feet hurt a lot right then, and they were very swollen. Before I could say anything, I just barked, "Stop it!" the way I would say it to Amber if he bit me. I was blown away. This person I scarcely know comes walking into my bedroom, touching me. I could have strangled her on the spot. She got a little sheepish and said, "I'll, I'll call you." I have decided she is not coming in this house. She is poison. It's all about her and whatever it is she needs. I am just not in the business of supplying that now.

RM: Sure, I think that's right. What an invasion of your privacy!

N: That was so intrusive, and I just do not have the resilience for it. It was one of the most memorable talks that Pat and I have ever had. It did not need to be disfigured by this kind of intrusion. This was dramatic. It was so quick, too, which made it more dramatic. It really caught me off stride.

RM: Very upsetting. You do not need that.

N: It upset me for a long time afterwards. I do not need it, and I am not doing her any good, whatever she thinks she may want from me. I think people as needy as she is do not actually get it. They do not get it by pulling it out of other people, and so I'm not doing her any favors to coddle. I'm not required to.

RM: Absolutely, I am with you. It's something I did not see clearly until now. There were inklings of this in your early encounters—that this was how things might shape up. Even at the first encounter, which was surprising to me, how quickly the discussion moved to the topic of death—

N: Yes!

Commentary: Nell had told me about a previous discussion with Kristin. It had moved fast—too fast in my judgment—toward the topic of dying, bypassing the necessary step of building a trusting relationship. While Nell is open to conversation about her own death, she does not like to dwell on it, and she can't sustain conversational intensity over long periods. Pushing content that the patient is not ready to engage is not helpful. Discussing our own death requires courage and a trusting relationship since the uncertainty of the future can provoke intense anxiety. It requires good judgment about when to nudge, when to invite, and when to let be. Good therapeutic conversation has a rhythm where two willing partners balance between leading and following.

RM: I have only known her professionally in her work with a friend who died in 1993. Kristin helped with her care in her last days. That's how she came to mind as we were contemplating hospice care. I am sorry that it came to that kind of unpleasant interaction. You do not need that.

N: I do not need it. I do not want to make trouble, but it's good that you understand how there are many caregivers who are in this work out of their own deep needs. I think she is one of them.

RM: I think you are right. You have a well-tuned BS detector.

Commentary: What happened between Nell and Kristin illustrates three important issues in caregiving including, most importantly, a physical and emotional boundary violation. First, the professional caregiver's needs and schedule conflicted with the patient's. Second, the interaction interrupted Nell's conversation with a valued friend, and third, it included a physical boundary violation—tickling Nell's feet. It precluded what I had hoped would be a helpful relationship with an experienced nurse who shares Nell's faith tradition. I felt badly; I hated seeing Nell upset and by a person I brought to her. I cringed when I heard her account of the interaction. The imbalance of power in relationships with bedridden patients can be a problem.

Nell as patient is at the mercy of whoever visits since she cannot be the gatekeeper to her home. Al is a kind, gentle soul, who would turn away no one he thought would be helpful to Nell.

N: This is my bedroom! I mean, there is something really so fundamentally asymmetrical about being in your nightgown in the last ditch of privacy in the bedroom of your home, and people can come and go and come and go. You are always at risk for becoming an object. The risk of this will increase with more professionals coming. When someone abuses it, you just get upset.

RM: You've got strong fire in you! That's good.

N: I do! My psychological state is active! Do not tickle my feet— not unless I ask you to (laughs).

RM: OK. (Laughs.) Are your feet hurting?

N: No. Anna was here today and gave me a massage. I sat up for about an hour on my computer typing and learned that sitting up is bad for my feet. The circulation has gotten demented down there. They are painful. It can't be helped, and I know that. We have been working on it. Hospice sent their chaplain in yesterday. Audrey suggested they come, and I thought it can't hurt and might help. She was very nice. King James version of the Bible, but very nice and not so doctrinaire. Very much of the persuasion that death is a mystery, and all we can do is trust. She talked very much about faith as the kind of bedrock of trust. She was talking about faith and God. It is hard to pull out of my mind certain notions of God because I am always translating the deity. I do not get along with he/she notions of a deity, so I am not sure of the chaplain's deity.

RM: I can relate to that.

N: (Laughs.) I am not sure deity is even what I'm reaching for. It is the life force or the love that makes the world go round—that fundamental thing that I'm trusting in, whatever it is. What she was really talking about was the promise that we will not be alone. It was good. I am trying to integrate the idea. That's what the dream was about—trying to integrate living and dying. The waking up was an epiphany, which is why I want the epiphany to be part of our dialogue.

RM: The email you sent explaining your dream and epiphany was beautiful.

Commentary: In Chapter 3, Nell described a dream about pure love waiting on the other side of her death. It was a great comfort to her. She did not go into detail about it then. She now wants to ensure that we record the dream and her epiphany. Nell sent me an email after our discussion of her dream (Box 7.1). Then we returned to discussing her epiphany.

N: Wasn't it beautiful? I'm trying to learn. How you think from the top of your head, and it goes down and down and down, down, and it finally gets into your bones. Then I really know it, and I keep trying to learn to trust.

RM: It's a lifelong task—learning to trust, who to allow into your room, into your head, and into your heart. Yes, you're still practicing. Me, too.

N: And specifically at the moment of death, I'm trying to practice trusting. What she [the chaplain] said was the only thing you can trust is that you will not be alone. That seems honest.

RM: Yes, you do have real live angels moving around you here on earth, including a noble guardian in Al. You feel it strongly, his watching over you, that you are not alone?

N: Yes, yes! It is a joy. I have arrived at a very peaceful place.

Commentary: I am both pleased about, and wary of, Nell's confidence in a peaceful dying. Things can go wrong in the end. I hope I can help her achieve her goal.

Box 7.1 Nell's Eiphany

I realized that in telling you about my early morning epiphany, I left out a key detail—how it began. It began, of course, with waking, but when I awoke, I was hearing a song, a hymn so beloved of my beloved Aunt Louise that it always evokes her. Since she died, about nine years ago, the advent of that song to my consciousness has always been a sign of her, of her emotional presence, and a remembrance of her goodness to me. The hymn isn't one we know (she was Presbyterian), but I know many of the words because she loved them:

Great Is Thy Faithfulness

Great is thy faithfulness, O God, my father,
There is no shadow of turning with thee.
Thou changest not, thy compassion it fails not.
Great is thy faithfulness, Lord unto me.
Pardon from sin and a peace that endureth,
Thy own dear presence to steer and to guide,
Strength for today, and bright hope for tomorrow,
Blessings all mine, with ten-thousand beside.

Refrain:
Great is thy faithfulness, great is thy faithfulness.
Morning by morning new mercies I see.
All I have needed thy hand hath provided.
Great is thy faithfulness, Lord unto me.

I think I've got it somewhat jumbled, but I'm sure you get the drift. It is a hymn of reassurance, and of thanksgiving; it suited perfectly the meaning and content of Fr. Jay's absolution and anointing, and I took it as a reiteration of the promise of the sacrament, and as a sign of the welcoming love of my "second mother." Both ways, it was a wonderful gift.

Then this concluding paragraph (slightly abridged) of Chapter 2, p. 20 of *My Ántonia* by Willa Cather came to me:

> I sat down in the middle of the garden . . . and leaned my back against a warm yellow pumpkin. . . . All about me giant grasshoppers, twice as big as any I had ever seen, were doing acrobatic feats among the dried vines. The gophers scurried up and down the ploughed ground. There in the sheltered draw-bottom the wind did not blow very hard, but I could hear it singing its humming tune up on the level, and I could see the tall grasses wave. The earth was warm under me, and warm as I crumbled it through my fingers. Queer little red bugs came out and moved in slow squadrons around me. Their backs were polished vermilion, with black spots. I kept as still as I could. Nothing happened. I did not expect anything to happen. I was something that lay under the sun and felt it, like the pumpkins, and I did not want to be anything more. I was entirely happy. Perhaps we feel like that when we die and become a part of something entire, whether it is sun and air, or goodness and knowledge. At any rate, that is happiness: to be dissolved into something complete and great. When it comes to one, it comes as naturally as sleep.

Dick, I think that the passage and the epiphany are related. That is why I emphasized those few sentences at the center of the Willa Cather passage. During what I'm calling my epiphany I felt perfectly free, without need or appetite. "I was entirely happy," and I realized consciously both (1) a strong, distinct reassurance that the moment of dying that has so haunted me will, when it comes, be as peaceful as the moment in which I then found myself, and (2) that I was free to go or stay now. I think I could have lain down again and not awakened. However, I realized that I have not finished living. My sister says that I will die when my spirit is willing to let go, and maybe she's right. But I think that only my body will let me go, because my pleasure in the scent of the air and the shifting patterns of the clouds—not to mention all the delights of family and friends—is so great that I keep coming back for more.

RM: You are planning well. Some of this you trust to others; some people you trust more. You have Audrey, the chaplain, Anna, Pat, me, Sally, and possibly even more people in the evening, if you want them. If you become less alert, you might want to have somebody in addition to Al here by your side.

N: Right now, I'm feeling alert for the moment. We have a very successful kind of structure to the evenings with our little sandwich and two hours of television. Then it's time to read a bit in bed, and then I am really zonked. That makes it very companionable, low-key, manageable, and supportive.

RM: You're talking about three, four hours in the evening?

N: Yes. That's a big stretch of time for me.

RM: Of course. During the day you have some people coming in, too?

N: Sally's here most of the time when Al's not here. I talked with Al. He used to go down for lunch. It meant that all morning, I was alone. Now I have asked him to eat breakfast upstairs when I'm asleep. I do not want to be alone when I sleep. Al goes down for exercises, but the tradeoff is that I can get up if I have to. Now I want to be sure that we debrief completely on Kristin.

RM: Yes. She was aware of what you described. I do not think she was aware of how strongly you felt, but she was aware of the tension.

N: What did she say in her words?

RM: She spoke of your impatience and irritation with her.

N: She said to me, "Well, I wasn't able to concentrate when I wrote down the time, so I didn't get the time right, and I sort of thought, was it 2 or 3 or 3 to 4? I'll split the difference. I'll come at 3." I thought, "You called me! If you can't call me at a time when you can concentrate enough to write down what you've just gotten, which is the answer to your question, 'When can I come?', then please call me when your mind is free."

RM: You're right.

N: You know, I did not ask for this. It was the pushing. I think if she had not tried to push it off, as if it wasn't her fault, I would not have been so annoyed, but I just thought, "This really is not functional stuff here."

RM: You are clear—you have boundaries. You are able to describe them and tell people what your needs are. That is healthy. I like the notion of debriefing now to cleanse yourself as best you can of whatever toxic fumes entered your space.

N: It's very fragile here. Things are very finely tuned at this point. How could they not be? You are so right: *Detoxification* is the word for this debriefing.

RM: Anything else about debriefing your time with Kristin?

N: No. Thank you. It's a relief to shed that burden. What about your thoughts on Audrey?

RM: I understand what you sense. She is a young person—no extensive experience but confident and caring and competent about the work. She has an understanding of your psychological task here, perhaps more so than I expected regarding the psychological dimension and maybe a little less so with regard to medical intervention when needed.

N: That makes me nervous with her. I think she is not a planner.

RM: Her planning skill is not clear to me. Audrey would be the person to initiate help if she was here, and you thought you couldn't get your breath, and hospice would be the people to call.

N: I think the nurse on duty, whoever, would help. I would alert Al.

RM: OK. Three weeks ago, when you didn't have oxygen, I thought you were approaching a point where you needed more help. Since starting on oxygen, your energy level has improved. You are a different person, even though you have periods where you get fatigued.

N: I took the oxygen back to 2.8 liters, and then yesterday, I put it back up to about a little over three because I found after a few days, I wanted more oxygen, but I have not felt the need to push it any further. I agree it makes such a difference, especially sleeping.

RM: Good. That's going well—the sense of not being able to get your breath or not being able to swallow—those problems are gone?

N: They are pretty nearly fixed. The night before last, I got into bed and could not swallow. Just like a child, I went through all of our steps—what you taught me—and it worked. I sat up and waited, took a deep breath; I drank my water and felt better.

RM: Great.

N: OK, we've gone through the two people you talked with, and you talked with Pat as well. That was very helpful to her.

RM: Your dear friend Pat loves you.

N: She does, and I love her, too.

RM: She wants to be by your side here, and yet she is going to California. She's afraid you will die on her. I think you will be on earth when she returns.

N: I think so, too. Because I have my other task to do with our conversations. I can't possibly die right now until it's done. (Laughs.)

RM: (Laughs.) Right. I am with you.

N: I decided I'm going to write Fr. Bob a letter about my funeral liturgy, the service. See whether I can change the gospel for my liturgy to the Magnificat. Wouldn't that be neat? I think that would be very cool. Do you have a copy of the liturgy plan I wrote up?

RM: No, I don't. I can see what you have here. It's beautiful. Can I keep this?

N: Yes. And that's just some writings I've kept close for 20-odd years since Rahner died.[1] You can have them for your inspiration file.

RM: Thank you. Have you spoken to Fr. Bob about your funeral Mass plan?

N: Not recently, but I did that more than a year ago when I was first diagnosed.

Commentary: Funeral planning is a delicate matter. Some patients attribute nonexistent predictive knowledge to the healthcare provider, assuming that agreeing to discuss funeral plans is tantamount to acknowledging they will be dead soon. When I enter into this type of planning discussion with patients or caregivers, I explain that it's a good idea if the thought of planning is intrusive. Once it's done, they can focus on living. The patient often has to initiate this conversation with family who are reluctant to face mortality.

RM: You were jumping the gun back then, rolling out your casket too soon.

N: Well, you know, they thought I was bouncing right out of this world. That was the impression that I certainly got from my oncologist, whose name escapes me now. I had the impression of only months to live last spring, so it was at that time that I did this.

RM: Which was about one year ago.

N: Well, I remember it calculating out to be June of last year! I would die in June, roughly, was what I took away from her after all our treatments failed, and the tumor went galloping free all the way across the torso. She felt that we were in the "months" range. I think that was what she said, so I stopped doing chemotherapy. We had been doing chemo for about six months. Then we stopped for five months, so right about then is when I did the liturgy planning and the funeral home planning, so it would be done. Pat went with Al and me to Hayworth Miller. Pat is prepared. She is very experienced and talented at managing people and so forth. She will be good to troubleshoot all the little details for the family.

RM: Good planning.

N: I wanted Pat in on the funeral planning at Hayworth Miller, so she would be on the same page with Fr. Bob and the organist. I need to write to him, too, and ask for this change in the gospel because I wasn't very interested in the gospels right then. I was much more interested in the Psalms and Isaiah, so I had the shortest gospel practically on record. (Laughs.) Lately, in my imagery work with my dear friend Mary, Mary the mother of Jesus, came to the fore very much as a spirit guide to me. I really love that canticle, and if it's permitted for a canticle to be the gospel, why not?

RM: Of course.

N: You said you wanted to talk with me about someone.

RM: Yes. Last Thursday, I went to a workshop in Greensboro given by Therese Schroeder-Sheker.

N: Sounds like a story.

RM: There is a story to tell. She's a trained contemplative Benedictine who has created the Chalice of Repose Project. She presented a daylong workshop called Prescriptive Music in Palliative Care.[2] She is a concert-caliber harpist who plays at the bedside of dying people. That is what the Chalice of Repose Project is about, partly.

N: Wow!

RM: She has a training program associated with Catholic University of America in DC, School of Nursing, School of Music, and School of Social Work. They train people to play the harp at the beside. I went to the workshop thinking of you. I thought it would be wonderful if she could be at your side playing her beautiful music.

N: Sounds like it would be beautiful. How would such a miracle come about?

RM: It would be nearly a miracle. She lives in Mt. Angel, Oregon!

N: That *would* be a miracle. (Laughs.) However, there are recordings of her, aren't there? I would love it!

Commentary: *Attending Therese Schroeder-Sheker's workshop was timely, as Nell is now finding music especially soothing. I spoke with Therese about Nell and ordered the CD* Rosa Mystica. *When it arrived, Nell began playing it as she dozed off at night. She loved the Chalice of Repose Project and its mission: to lovingly care for the physical and spiritual needs of the dying with prescriptive music; to enable and to model a blessed, peaceful, conscious death; and to integrate contemplative values into daily life. Nell is actively contemplating her hoped-for peaceful death and using music to soothe her on the journey.*

RM: She taught me that there is something special about the person and the harp together. It's not just the harp; it's mostly about the person. The harp is a beautiful instrument, but it must have an empty chamber in order to make music. Human beings, in order to be fully alive, must have some place of emptiness, a place of contemplation and silence. She spoke about the strings that are anchored in the empty part of the harp.

N: Down in the wood.

RM: The harp sounds are seeking the heavens. In addition, it is only through the tension that you can get music. If there's no tension involved, if there's no emptiness, there is no music. She said it much more eloquently than I am. The message was beautiful. Likewise, if there is no emptiness, no tension in the person, how can you reach for the heavens? I thought, "This is the person who could sanctify and bring grace to your place of holiness, right here."

N: Isn't that dear of you—the Chalice of Repose Project.

RM: I know some harpists in town, but I don't know anybody that I would want to invite into your space just now. Therese Schroeder-Sheker is very special. You would resonate with the qualities that she brings to the bedside. She is a person of great depth. I ordered CDs from her.

N: Thank you. Anna has been bringing over music—I am getting so deliciously spoiled— beautiful Mozart quartets and wonderful arias. I just love the music.

RM: Music is healing.

N: Yes, it is! (Pointing) At the end of the table, under the gong, there should be a book with a red cover called *Journeying East*. It says that it's for you. I thought you could have it now.

RM: Thank you.

N: You probably don't need *Arrested in Kathmandu*, so I'll pass that on to Anna, but that one piece in the red book is about the man at the Zen Hospice Center in San Francisco—that's the one that I think is indispensable.

RM: This is a precious gift to me—a book with an article by the author whose name I can't pronounce.

N: (Chuckles.) Just for your sake, I am going to pronounce his name into the record here: Frank Ostaseski. His article is titled "Living and Dying Each Day."[3] He is with the Zen Hospice project, the first Buddhist hospice in the United States. You are sure to like this. (Laughs.)

RM: Thank you. I remember when you first brought this out to show me. It was some months ago, remember?

N: Yes.

RM: Thank you—this is precious. Now, in just a few minutes, you might want to rest a bit. Is there anything else on your mind tonight?

N: I certainly feel like I need help to be alert about this next level of care. I do not know when to lay it on, and I don't know with what person—whether it should be an RN or CNA or an LPN. Can you help me with that?

RM: You may be able to choose from a CNA, LPN, or RN. You probably do not need complete RN care now. I am going to leave the Bayada Nurses number. You might talk with Audrey about it as well. Call Bayada and ask them to do an assessment with you.

N: OK. Bayada Nurses. In addition, I should talk with Audrey, who's going to come tomorrow about this?

RM: Yes. Get her input, tell her what you are thinking—that in the evening and during the night, you might need someone to look after you. Are you getting up, going to the bathroom, and walking around?

N: I got a nightlight yesterday. Sally got it for me, and that's a help. My problems are accelerating incontinence. I just do not get to the bathroom in time anymore, but that's OK—I can accept that—because I am still able to get there.

RM: OK.

N: And it never yet has been out of my reach to get something I need. I am able to stand up. It could be my stubbornness.

RM: Stubbornness is good. There may be a need for something like Depends underwear?

N: Oh, I use something like Depends now because it just makes sense. Then I'm not worried about secondary things. It just makes cleanup easier. (Laughs.)

RM: You are doing great with the mechanics of body change as well as the transcendent. Being stuck on the earth, on the one hand, yet you can look out that window and see clouds—the vapor that we all become. At once flesh and feces and, on the other hand, air, vapor. This must be a funny god—a good sense of humor, perhaps?

N: I don't know. Does every god have so peculiar a sense of humor!? (Laughs.)

RM: (Laughs.) You've given me a good book to read and these wonderful gifts on the liturgy, Rahner, epiphany redone, your editing of our conversation regarding mortality. Thank you. Now I have a poem for you. Then I will be gone. Until next week.

N: All right. Ready (Box 7.2).

N: Beautiful.

RM: See you next week.

Final Commentary: This poem is an invitation to address despair, a feeling Nell disclosed at our first meeting. It touches on two prominent themes in our dialogues over the months. The first is loneliness. Nell has not left her apartment for several months. Her world is becoming smaller due to her physical decline. She is now relying more on her circle of friends, family, and new professionals to help her navigate

---

Box 7.2 Wild Geese

Mary Oliver

> You do not have to be good.
> You do not have to walk on your knees
> for a hundred miles through the desert repenting.
> You only have to let the soft animal of your body
> love what it loves.
> Tell me about despair, yours, and I will tell you mine.
> Meanwhile the world goes on.
> Meanwhile the sun and the clear pebbles of the rain
> are moving across the landscapes,
> over the prairies and the deep trees,
> the mountains and the rivers.
> Meanwhile the wild geese, high in the clean blue air,
> are heading home again.
> Whoever you are, no matter how lonely,
> the world offers itself to your imagination,
> calls to you like the wild geese, harsh and exciting—
> over and over announcing your place
> in the family of things.

the day. She is less interested in the wider world as reflected by the New York Times *and National Public Radio.*

The second theme is the idea that we are part of a larger family, "the family of things." Nell is strongly communal and recognizes her place in the larger world, just like Mary Oliver, who so eloquently speaks of the connection between nature and humans. Nell's connections have become more localized, centering on what she can see and hear from her apartment and the people she interacts with in person and via phone and email. Her circle of involvement is becoming much smaller due to physical limitations and lack of emotional and energy reserves. However, her circle of concern remains large as she sees the connection between all things.

The poem "Wild Geese"[4] provides soothing words to end our conversation. As Nell becomes more comfortable with her dying, she becomes more content with her living, a surprising twist she names in our next conversation.

Notes

1. Karl Rahner (1904–1984) was a German Jesuit priest considered one of the most influential Roman Catholic theologians of the 20th century. He believed that we act from, and respond to, God's grace, as fully manifest in the life of Jesus, when we demonstrate an absolute love for our neighbors, readiness for death, and hope for the future. See Rahner, K. (1978). *Foundations of Christian faith: An introduction to the idea of Christianity* (W. B. Dych, Trans.). New York: Seabury Press; and Michaud, D. (n.d.). Karl Rahner (1904–1984). In W. Wildman (Ed.), *Boston collaborative encyclopedia of Western Theology*. Boston: Boston University. http://people. bu.edu/wwildman/bce/rahner.htm

2. The Chalice of Repose Project describes prescriptive music as a compound sonic medicine delivered live, at the bedside, on polyphonic instruments, by practitioners certified in music-thanatology by the Chalice of Repose Project. Using voice and harp, musician-clinicians can work in teams of two, positioning themselves on either side of the dying patient. The person who is receiving the music may be experiencing either physiological pain or

interior suffering or both, and may be morphine-intolerant, needing non-invasive and nonmechanical, profoundly human responses to increasing vulnerability. In all cases, the musician-clinician is working with vital signs and is able to document in an evidence-based medicine the physiology of pain relief. Additional information can be found on their website: https://chaliceofrepose.org/

3. Ostaseski, F. (2000). *The five invitations: Discovering what death can teach us about living fully.* New York: Flatiron Books. The five invitations or five gifts are (1) don't wait; (2) welcome everything; push away nothing; (3) bring your whole self to the experience; (4) find a place of rest in the middle of things; and (5) cultivate "don't-know" mind, by which he means a mind that is open and receptive.

4. Oliver, M. (1986). *Dream work.* (p. 14) New York: Atlantic Monthly Press.

8

May 17, 2005—Acceptance

Today is not the day

I can't just sit here
staring death in her face
blinking and asking for a new name
by which to greet her

I am not afraid to say
unembellished
I am dying
but I do not want to do it
looking the other way.

Lorde, A. (1993). *The marvelous arithmetics of distance: Poems 1987–1992.* (p. 57) New York: W. W. Norton & Company.

Main Themes: Accepting well-being and happiness while welcoming death, letting go of friends; finding humor in an online nightgown purchase that may not arrive in time.

Nell's main unfinished task is dying. She is impatient with her stay in mortal time although getting better at symptom management and finding meaning with husband Al. Her sense of well-being surprises her, and she wonders if it is an obstacle. She finds her situation—busy living while talking about dying—comic and paradoxical. She appreciates the irony of purchasing expensive nightgowns that may not arrive in time before she dies.

Nell begins the session by asking me to help her deliver gifts to the people she loves. The task of shedding her possessions and relationships has become more urgent now, yet letting go of the things that help us to remember who we are is no simple task. Nell is managing to detach from her objects, even though in contemporary America we are what we own.

Dialogue 8

N: I found that I have two very beautiful wall rugs from Nepal here. Could you carry them off to Dr. T?

RM: Yes, I can. What a wonderful gift!

N: I inherited them. They are beautiful. Just this week, I was going over with the consigner what was left from the house and learning about things that hadn't moved. I had forgotten all about them. I think Dr. T will be pleased.

RM: Yes, he will. Have you spoken to him?

N: Scheduled for Friday. I want to talk to you about it. Now, it has been eight weeks since I started with hospice with our "days-to-weeks" timeline. I was thinking that you have at least twice said there may be an unfinished task for me, though we don't know what it is. Would you say more about that?

RM: There *may* be a task to be finished. Since you are managing your physical symptoms so well, perhaps we should revise that days-to-weeks timeline? Now that you're on oxygen, there has been significant improvement in breathing. Your last lab readings were normal. Your organs are functioning well, including your liver, even though you have what you call this "anchor place" there—the bulging tumor.

Commentary: *Nell is referring to the phrase I used over eight weeks ago as a very rough measure of her possible life expectancy, given her tumor burden. When patients or family caregivers ask my medical oncology colleagues to predict expected lifespan, some use this time scale: hours-to-days, days-to-weeks, weeks-to-months, or months-to-years. Having a general idea can be comforting to people, particularly those who accept death as inevitable and want to finish their earthly business. This topic is of intense interest in medical oncology.*[1] *I asked one of my physician colleagues how she helps her patients when they press her for an answer. She begins by explaining the uncertainty of prediction and, if pressed further, selects what she deems the appropriate duration from the time scale referred to here. The new immunotherapy drugs render accurate prediction even more problematic.*

N: The last few days, I have been experiencing a sense of well-being. I'm interested in exploring this. Typically, I am very limited on things like sitting up or eating. I continue to lose weight. There is some limit to what the body will give me, but it does not seem to have reached that limit yet. Isn't that amazing?

RM: It is amazing. You have a sense of well-being. Tell me more about that.

N: Last night, I was thinking, "What is the task that I could have left undone?" I was thinking that one of the things that is holding me here is that Al and I are so happy. I felt that when the three of us were talking. That was really nice two weeks ago, at our last meeting. I think you called it "the great forgiveness." It relieves me enormously of all that baggage.

RM: Yes.

N: I do not push or expect things from him that aren't realistic. I just enjoy what is there, and we just enjoy being together. I am not holding on to crap.

Commentary: Nell has forgiven Al and moved on to achieve a new level of intimate conversation and shared experience with him. Their busy life prior to cancer left little space for closeness, but Nell's diagnosis set in motion a search for deeper emotional connection, which she has now reestablished with Al. Many cancer patients feel a sense of isolation, which can be especially acute if intimate emotional connection has been missing in their primary relationship.

RM: Yes, old baggage to deal with or even enjoying life could keep you here.

N: Do you think that?

RM: Yes. What's keeping you here does not have to be bad. Being content and happy on earth does not have to be an obstacle to leaving, either.

N: I guess that's part of the question, isn't it? There's nothing wrong with living. It's keeping me here on earth. (Laughs.)

RM: There's nothing wrong with your life. I know you have been preparing to die for a long time. At one point in our conversation, you had talked about being 16 months alive after your first "sentence" of an expiration date of about eight months! Now your second "sentence" had to do with our talk of living days-to-weeks two months ago. Perhaps we should have been talking weeks-to-months at that point?

N: It certainly seemed very reasonable at the time and still does now because there is some floor below which I can't give. But you're saying that with the latest labs, I don't seem to be near there now?

RM: Yes, that's right. You're eating, drinking milkshakes, and you're up, enjoying life. You have a sense of well-being. And you are telling me there is some floor, some lowering of your functioning, that you know can't go much lower?

N: Yes.

RM: I don't believe there is magic about a particular task being accomplished and then all of a sudden, you drop off. It seems rather than losing tasks, you've actually added a task—our dialogues and your work with them. I'd like to hear if you think our talks are an obstacle to you. Are our conversations keeping you here?

N: Our dialogues? Oh no, oh no, not at all! I wish I had more to contribute.

RM: Your contributions are the core. There is so much richness in our conversation. Your words will last for a long time. I am riding on your wings.

N: It is collaboration.

RM: It is, and you are teaching about one of life's most important lessons—how to let go.

N: This is an unexpected route, a joyous one—to turn corner after corner after corner, now temporarily reaching a plateau of satisfaction.

RM: Yes, uh-huh. That's beautiful.

N: It is grace. It did not come until I had reached and maintained for some days a kind of acceptance. Not total—I doubt that anyone totally embraces the idea of their own death. We cannot embrace the idea of our own death because we cannot apprehend it totally. Having reached as far as I can go with the idea of my own death, I see that my situation is taught in the universe by whatever we mean when we say God. It was not until I had gotten there that I could then say that, "Oh, I do accept mortality, my ending, and I'm happy."

RM: You have been courageous in facing into this process— physical, spiritual, emotional—right from the first time we met and you said, "The problem is despair."

N: Now the despair is gone. Coming back to what we were saying about conversation, another cause for my well-being is that, paradoxically, I have cut off a fair amount of conversation. I've just sent emails to a number of people who telephone a lot and asked them to stick to email. The telephone is a difficult instrument now to work with. It's hard to hear with the rushing of the oxygen in my ears. It's hard to talk, sit up, and especially hard to generate the focus on the other person, when the other person is just a voice in your ear. Several phone calls per day are just overwhelming. I have just cut the phone out practically, except to be tucked in by phone. I love to be talking on the phone just before closing my eyes to sleep. (Laughs.)

RM: Good idea.

N: My friends want to call and want to be in touch. They want to express concern, but they don't know what to say. They hang on the phone and tell me about their children, what plays they've just seen, or whatever. I have said, "Please don't do that anymore." In a way, paradoxically, cutting out some conversations allows me to be more present. I feel the need to be present to myself spiritually now in the way that I haven't felt for several weeks. I just feel the need to cocoon.

RM: That's a beautiful word, *cocoon*. I have a poem by Lynn Felder I will give to you titled "Cocooning" (Box 8.1).[2] You will like it. Say more about your cocooning.

N: Well, I'm not sure really. It's partly prayer; it's partly just being open to new questions like asking myself, "What is wrong with being alive, if I'm doing so well at being alive?" (Laughs.) You remember, I juggled with the notion that it was my task to finish this dying process, but what if it's not yet my task? Right now, it's my task to continue this living process.

RM: You look very much alive to me.

N: It's all right with me. (Laughs.) Part of cocooning is just leaving the time to ask questions like that.

Commentary: Nell has managed her symptoms of pain and discomfort, so living each day is no longer an ordeal. While she has renewed energy, she is nevertheless tightening her circle of involvement by cutting back on daily telephone contact with friends and limiting her time with National Public Radio and the New York Times. *This process is taking place in fits and starts over a period of weeks.*

RM: That is beautiful. When you told me your sister Ruth said, "You will leave when your spirit's ready," I thought, "Your spirit's fine. It's your body that's not ready." You have been roaming in the world of the living and the dying for a while, but your body is not ready.

N: I bribed my body. I asked my friend Pat to hustle me up two cotton summer nightgowns, ordered last Friday. (Laughs.)

RM: Nice.

Box 8.1   Cocooning

Lynn Felder

Winter came slow that year:
Summer lasted till December.
Then the cold came down
Like a cocoon,
Wrapping us in blades of silver,
Zissing down in icedrops,
Gathering us in.

I was ill and frightened,
A secret sickness in my belly
Like an alien baby
 Or a tiny ticking bomb.

I lay in my warm bed,
The alien gone,
The bomb still ticking,
And dreamed of death and life and birth
And what I had been
And what I would and would not be.
The cold
Gathered us in
And I lay in my warm bed,
Thinking the winter
Was a good time to be sick,
Time to breathe and gather and flow,
Time to be in a warm bed
And dream of hummingbirds and eagles
And the fierce white light of hope and heaven

And the illimitable possibilities of living and dying.
Outside the bare limbs creak and groan.
Sometimes the earth must lose everything
Before it can bloom and live again.

I lie in my warm bed
And breathe and dream and flow,
Meditate into a soft belly
That does not resist god's love
Or the illimitable possibilities of living and dying.
The body is just a body—like a cocoon.
It is the heart that wants healing.
It is the heart that can change color,
Grow wings
    And learn to dance.

N: And they need to be cotton but lighter weight than these. There are two of these and then a third one like them, so I can keep them ironed. Pat went off and came back with two that didn't fit, and so I wrote her an email and said, "That's OK—I'll go online and look." I went online and naturally, I found the most luscious, expensive, gorgeous, perfect answers—$150 apiece! (Laughs.)

RM: Wonderful.

N: I ordered them. I have never done anything like that. Dick, it was so funny because then it was complete and online, so you can never undo it. Then I was completely overwhelmed with trepidation. Who spends $150 on a nightgown? Who does that? (Laughs.)

RM: Nell does that. You were horrified with yourself. (Laughs.)

N: I was horrified with myself and kept this secret for about a day and a half. Finally, I marched in here and said to myself, "Well,

it's OK!" While I was being horrified, I began wondering—
what if I don't live long enough, and they arrive after I've died?
I put them on a two–three-day delivery, but it was Friday, and
those were business days, so they'll probably come tomorrow.
What if they arrive, and I'm not here to explain? Then the Visa
bill comes, and Al is looking at it and saying, "What is this?
I have no idea what this is. Oh my dear, late-lamented Nell!
What did she do?" (Laughs.)

RM: You know the answer to that, don't you? You can't die until you
get those gowns!

N: Exactly! I was on the horns of a dilemma, so I marched Al in and
asked him to sit down. I told him I had a confession to make.
I showed him the print of the invoice from online and explained
that I had done this thing, and he of course thought that was just
fine. I slept better. Until then, I was dreaming that it was a secret.
I was dreaming about them all night. They still haven't come, so
that's probably another reason that I'm still alive. (Laughs.)

RM: Well, it's just Tuesday, and you are very much alive!

N: That's right!

Commentary: *Even with death near, Nell can laugh at herself and her
potential predicament—dying and leaving Al with a surprise bill. She
would not dream of ordering a $150 nightgown except on her deathbed.*

RM: Your color is good. Your spirit is strong. We'll know Friday
about your labs. You have lots of time for those gowns.

N: When I was rationalizing about buying them, I thought that
when they sent me home from the clinic on hospice care, and
Dr. T was saying days-to-weeks, I was thinking the end was
very near, and that did not happen. Remember?

RM: Yes, I do. You have been full of surprises, Nell. You might be
ordering tomato plants before long!

N: Tomatoes?

RM: Tomato plants. They ripen in July.

N: That is an exquisite possibility. Imagine the logistics of getting someone to come plant tomatoes. (Laughs.)

RM: Dr. T said a while back that it was time for hospice, and you were thinking, "Whoa there! That seems too soon." That was about two months ago.

N: That's right. That was when I said my goal was not to call hospice until the last minute because I did not want to be in their care until it was time, and there was no alternative. He said, "The time is now." He was very clear.

RM: Yes.

N: So once again—

RM: You confound—

N: Expectations.

RM: Expectations. The prognosticators and their predictions. You have been doing it all along.

N: Now I have two nightgowns to explain! (Laughs.)

RM: You're like Mark Twain: The rumors of your death are an exaggeration!

N: Yes, greatly exaggerated! However, I do think that cutting down on food matters. I eat half of what I ate two to three weeks ago. That's helpful because it goes down better, and it stays down. I don't have so many troubles. I'm also cutting down on the obligatory socialness with people, conserving energy.

RM: You are adapting, living your life with zest, integrity, thoughtfulness. Some relationships are beginning to fall away. The phone as a way for connecting to people is falling away. There may not necessarily be a task to accomplish or words you need to speak to anyone. I want you to know how much I appreciate you, your courage, and our relationship. You are very special to me.

N: And you to me, too.

RM: You are a source of inspiration, faith, and trust. I want to make sure that your message is heard through our recorded conversation.

N: Thank you. It means a lot to me, too, even though I do not feel like I have anything to say.

RM: You have much to say, so much to give—you have already given words. Your message is still emerging. I hope it will be echoing for many years to come.

N: I hope so, too.

RM: There may not be a certain thing for you to do or say that is keeping you here. Perhaps just being open to the transcendent is enough now. Then there's the body—pain meds, labs, food, oxygen. In those areas, are you getting what you need from hospice, Al, or Sally?

N: Yes. Pat gave me a back rub yesterday.

RM: Great.

N: That was wonderful because being in bed all the time, my back at this point is very sore, very tender. Cramps up, you know. All around the middle, from my shoulder blades down to my waist, it cramps up a lot, and she just did such a nice job. That was a first massage, but I think there will soon be a second. (Laughs.)

RM: That's wonderful. I know Pat was with you Friday. She comes to visit and can give you a massage.

N: Yes, Anna came today for several hours so that Al could be on campus.

RM: It's good that you can organize, so Al can get out. You feel OK about being here without him, and Al feels OK about leaving?

N: Yes, very nice. Now that school is over, and that activity is not there for him, I am going to encourage him to go ahead and ask his driver to do errands, do things that he cares about. Go to the drugstore and the bank and get his hair cut and stuff. He can do that.

RM: You are doing a great job organizing.

N: Al has really changed a lot. He is much more gregarious. I think it's being here and with people.

RM: Yes, you have been doing a lot of teaching with Al, too. You thought you left your teaching job behind. (Laughs.) The lesson plans are spontaneously created!

N: They are. Very spontaneously created. (Laughs.)

RM: Are you feeling tired right now?

N: Very sleepy, for some reason. I'm sorry to say I feel very sleepy. How long have we been talking?

RM: It is just now 7:00 PM. You're all talked out. Do you want to hear a poem?

N: I would love to hear a poem or two. When you have read the poem, I'll show you the rugs.

RM: OK. The poem is "In a Dark Time" by Theodore Roethke.[3] The first stanza was in a book written by Barbara Sourkes called *The Deepening Shade*.[4] We have used this with graduate students doing a placement in our Cancer Patient Support and Psychosocial Oncology Programs. I love the imagery—the deepening shade, which, in our setting, in Cancerland, refers to the experience of the diagnosis and treatment of cancer. Sourkes is using Roethke's imagery to describe the psychological experience of cancer (Box 8.2).

RM: It's full of wisdom.

N: It brings to mind the canticle of Zachariah that begins in the middle of his life. It reminded me of how Dante begins *The Divine Comedy*: "In the middle of my life, I awoke in a dark wood." The whole journey of *The Divine Comedy* takes place in the middle of his life as a realization: "In the middle of the journey of our life, I found myself astray in a dark wood where the straight road had been lost sight of." Yes. And now we can look at those rugs.

Final Commentary: The poem by Roethke has special meaning for me as a therapist who has spent his professional career working in cancer care. I believe that the self—the eye or I Roethke refers to—is more visible in the darkness. It is through suffering we can encounter

Box 8.2 In a Dark Time

Theodore Roethke

In a dark time, the eye begins to see,
I meet my shadow in the deepening shade;
I hear my echo in the echoing wood—
A lord of nature weeping to a tree,
I live between the heron and the wren,
Beasts of the hill and serpents of the den.
What's madness but nobility of soul
At odds with circumstance? The day's on fire!
I know the purity of pure despair,
My shadow pinned against a sweating wall,
That place among the rocks—is it a cave,
Or winding path? The edge is what I have.
A steady storm of correspondences!
A night flowing with birds, a ragged moon,
And in broad day the midnight come again!
A man goes far to find out what he is—
Death of the self in a long, tearless night,
All natural shapes blazing unnatural light.
Dark, dark my light, and darker my desire.
My soul, like some heat-maddened summer fly,
Keeps buzzing at the sill. Which I is I?
A fallen man, I climb out of my fear.
The mind enters itself, and God the mind,
And one is One, free in the tearing wind.

our self, learn who we are in this world. Being near the suffering of
cancer patients over these many years has been a gift and a burden—
the gift of being close to courage; the burden of being close to pain and

suffering—the darkness. Nell is entering her own deepening shade as she approaches death with humor, curiosity, and an open heart. What she finds in her deepening shade is a surprise revealed in our next dialogue.

Notes

1. Epstein, A. S., Prigerson, H. G., O'Reilly, E. M., & Maciejewski, P. K. (2016). Discussions of life expectancy and changes in illness understanding in patients with advanced cancer. *Journal of Clinical Oncology, 34*(20), 2398–2403; Hagerty, R. G., Butow, P. N., Ellis, P. M., Lobb, E. A., Pendlebury, S. C., Leighl, N., MacLeod, C., & Tattersall, M. H. N. (2005). Communicating with realism and hope: Incurable cancer patients' views on the disclosure of prognosis. *Journal of Clinical Oncology, 23,* 1278–1288; Simone, C. B. (2016). Discordant expectations about prognosis in critically ill patients. *Annals of Palliative Medicine, 5*(3), 225–226.

2. Nell identifies the need to cocoon, which means "to envelop or surround protectively, insulate." She is retreating to the comfort of her home and the love of Al, family, and friends. Lynn Felder, a journalist, yoga instructor, and survivor of ovarian cancer, composed a poem about her cocooning (see Box 8.1). I gave the poem to Nell later.

3. Roethke, T. (1975). *The collected poems.* Garden City, NY: Doubleday.

4. Sourkes, B. (1982). *The deepening shade: Psychological aspects of life-threatening illness.* Pittsburgh: University of Pittsburgh Press.

9

May 24, 2005—Finding Home

The ache for home lives in all of us, the safe place where we
can go as we are and not be questioned.

> Angelou, M. (1986). *All God's children need
> traveling shoes* (p. 196). New York: Random House.

Main Themes: A spiritual crisis, fearing her faith is not complete,
letting go of friends, and finding a place called home.

Nell discusses the importance of faith and receiving the
Sacrament of Confession and the ritual of anointing the senses.
Through her brother John's dream of reuniting, she finally feels
what it is like to "go home," to return to feelings of family, even
when those feelings include recollection of violence, which Nell
wisely sees as preparation for death. At the same time, she is letting go of her family and friends by setting boundaries and closing
down phone calls and emails. Holding on and letting go, a fundamental rhythm of life, is shifting toward release. Nell's dear friend
Mary articulates this painful process and her hope of their reunion
in a beautiful card.

When loving family members or friends try to express compassion with cancer patients, it can feel like pity, e.g., "You poor thing,"
which irritates rather than comforts. In this peculiar dynamic, the
patient experiences the caregiver's good intention as overly solici-
tous. Nell experiences this and reports its effect on her. Misguided
attempts at compassion can create distance, not closeness.

When I arrived, Nell was reading a transcript from a previous conversation, preparing for our session.

Dialogue 9

RM: I see you've been working—editing our dialogues.

N: I was trying to get refreshed as to what we had said last week, but I wasn't making much progress. Do you recall what we said last week?

RM: We began with our normal checklist of topics, talked about body mechanics, the routines of medicine, lab tests. We talked about the life of the mind and the nightgowns. You were worried the nightgowns would come, and you would be gone. Al would be there with a bill. He wouldn't know what was going on. The nightgowns and a bill, but no Nell!

N: (Laughs.) Here's the nightgown.

RM: It's beautiful. You know, somehow I pictured red. I just imagined that you would have a beautiful red gown.

N: It's not red—red has been the toenails, not the gown. The toenails need daily care.

RM: Yes, of course. I have news for you. I talked with Therese Schroeder-Sheker, the contemplative harpist from Oregon. I told her about our conversations. You recall we spoke about her, wishing she could be here, at the bedside with you? I ordered her music weeks ago, but she had a tragedy in her family—her father died unexpectedly. She currently runs the music store and didn't have a chance to send the music out. I told her you liked classical and gospel music like the Shades of Praise group.[1] She's sending CDs in overnight mail.

N: Oh, how lovely! Thank you! That's very sad about her father.

RM: Yes, it is. She's managing. She described expansive music that might be helpful for you now.

N: I need it. I'm hanging on to the Bible, sleeping with a rosary and talking to those images of Mary and Jesus on the wall. I am generally trying to keep my soul tied down with anchors.

RM: Yes, for sure.

N: I had an interesting time with Fr. Bob. I asked him to hear my confession. I confessed my fear that my faith was not complete. I said if my faith was complete, I wouldn't be afraid. He said he didn't believe that was a sin. He didn't believe that anybody's faith was complete in that sense, which was helpful. I think he's right. Faith is the work of every day saying *yes*, and the yes is saying you're not alone. Would you like to look at my screensaver—and read it? It reassures me that I am not alone.

RM: Yes, I can read it: "The force of love gathers about you. You are in harmony and secure."

N: That came in an email from you.

RM: My God, I can make sense every now and then!

N: (Laughs.) Yes, you do good email. What you said is important.

RM: It's naming the truth. It's easy to do that.

N: No, it's not! It's hard to find the truth.

RM: You're seeking truth, aren't you?

N: Trying to stay there. Trying not to fall out of it.

RM: I appreciate your reflections on confession, and I like the response of the confessor on faith and fear. If Jesus can despair in the Garden of Gethsemane, probably humans can be afraid as well without being sinful. I respect you for naming your fear and searching for deeper faith to come from that fear.

N: Then he said, "Are you afraid of God?" I said, "No, I'm afraid of the moment of transition. I'm afraid it will hurt, and I'm afraid of violence." That word *violence*, I suddenly realized, was the core issue—exactly what I'm afraid of. I have dealt with a lot of violence. One blow with a strap is violent. (Pause. Tears.) When it happens again, it's like taking a needle in my chemo port without the anesthetic. Sometimes you have to take things like that. If that is all I'm afraid of, I've been there; I've endured that;

and I can do it again. There are payoffs to a rough childhood. (Chuckles through tears.)

RM: Take my hand. You have a wonderful sense of humor that shines in you even when facing fear—the fear of what violence can do, what it has done to you. The sound of the word and what it means are both frightening, yet you draw upon your childhood as a preparation for your ultimate adulthood transition. You are wise, dear Nell.

Commentary: Nell has spoken of her father's harsh discipline using a strap. Reconciling family conflict during her childhood and adolescence has been an intermittent theme throughout our conversations. Her life review revealed deep wounds and her capacity for forgiveness as well as letting go of bitterness as she nears the end of her rich life.

N: Thank you for being here. I would like to think I'll sleep away. For a long time, I assumed I would not sleep away. That was the problem. Then I realized I have to be prepared. I want it to sleep away, not meet violence again. Chances are that it will be that way from what people say.

RM: Yes.

N: I must accept whatever comes.

RM: I am with you on acceptance of what comes and seeing your way to peacefulness. You are there already. There are times when things are upsetting, like the delay in a response from hospice. You are more peaceful even with those things these days. You are maintaining your sense of humor and direction. You have a clear path toward the new world.

N: I finally feel what people call "going home."

RM: Yes, tell me about it.

N: I had the most wonderful email from my brother John, who wrote and said that he had had a vision. His back was hurting him a lot, so he lay down to take a nap. In that sleeping/waking time, he had a vision in which Jesus met him, took his hand, greeted him, and walked with him across the Jordan River. Waiting on the other side were our mother and me. He said we had so much catching up to do. He reflected on the vision. Only after he'd really awakened did he remember that our father is dead. Johnny really had a destructive symbiotic relationship with our daddy, and he said it felt natural that he was not there. He did not feel called to dwell on that. He loved the anticipation of love and the presence of the Lord, and he thanked me for being his sister. I was just blown away. I emailed him back and said the same.

RM: That's beautiful, Nell. Something touched him deeply. Something is stirring in his soul and his heart in relation to your great movement here. There is a bond between the two of you.

N: Yes, there always was. He is seven years younger than I am— he's always seven years younger than I am. (Laughs.) In the pairing of kids in the family, he was my pal. We always had a closer relationship than he or I had with any of the other kids.

Commentary: Throughout her adult life, Nell has felt more or less distant from her family. We have discussed this periodically over the past months. The metaphor of going home *expresses her return to her family, deeper understanding of her siblings, and reaching a sense of place and belonging in this world. It has been very gratifying and represents a final holding on and letting go of her brothers and sisters as she returns to the home of her soul.*

RM: You two have always been close?

N: Yes, just as my sister Ruth had that kind of closeness with my brother Walter.

RM: Have you been keeping in touch with Ruth by emails or calls as well?

N: Ruth—every other day or so. Walter is not so frequent, and I'm sure that's partly because I never write back. (Laughs.) But they're very busy. They have a 16-year-old, and her husband is on the road all the time, and Ruth works. They don't have much time to write.

RM: Have you told Ruth or Walter about your spiritual preparations?

N: No, I don't know them that well. Walter is 14 years younger than I am, and we just have been getting acquainted this year.

RM: Do they know that you're very ill?

N: Yes, they do, and they periodically send loving cards.

RM: And of course you've confounded every prediction.

N: (Laughs.) Well, yes, I have. On another topic, I want to thank you for asking Fr. Bob about the complete form of anointing.

RM: I told him of your hopes for anointing of all of the senses. He said that he had never anointed all the senses but would be open to it. So that was the first time you got the full senses treatment?

N: Yes, it was good. He said the ritual was discontinued before he was ordained, so he'd never anointed all the senses. He got a little legalistic—he said it's discontinued, but it's permitted. It's "listed," as it were. (Laughs.)

RM: All right, I won't report you. When you get a little closer to God, you can check these things out from the true source! (Both laugh.)

N: OK, I want to talk this out with you. I need to write to my friend Carol. I've been writing to people, but it's harder to keep it ongoing. Carol is the jellybeans friend who works for Commonweal. She's also the one who screams in my ear, "Oh, you poor baby! Oh, you lamb, you!" whenever she thinks about how sick I am. She calls me up to tell me how sick I am! It's gotten to the point where I cannot bear it anymore. I wrote her and said, "I love talking with you, and I love you, but it's increasingly difficult to talk on the phone, and I'd appreciate sticking to email and snail mail." She came back snippy, kind of, and said, "It wasn't easy to generate conversation anyway, so it's just as well." I thought, "I wasn't calling you—you were calling me!" (Laughs.)

RM: Yes, for sure.

Commentary: Nell identifies a problem many cancer patients experience. Loving family members or friends who attempt to express sympathy or empathy actually show pity. Pity can irritate rather than comfort, especially for someone like Nell, who is very independent. She cringes and wants to avoid it. One clinician calls compassion that may be overly dramatic and emotional "airhead compassion." Such contact creates distance rather than closeness. Paul Ricoeur makes a poignant distinction: To show compassion is to understand the "suffering with" that the word signifies: "It is not a moaning-with as pity, commiseration, figures of regret can be; it is a struggling with, an accompanying—if not sharing that identifies oneself with the other."[2]

N: But you know how people get—they want to be in touch; they want to make a difference. They can't make a difference, really. She was making it my problem, which it isn't. I just let it pass, and in a few days, she sent a nice email with a poem attached, so I knew she had gotten over it. Then I had to have the same talk with Mary.

RM: Your dear friend who does guided imagery?

N: Yes. She called night-before-last. She was just back from her trip, so she downloaded about the trip first, and then she started asking me all these probing questions about where I was, wanting to be reassured that I was still buoyed up by the work that we had done. It took the form of a series of questions, just relentless questions, to which yes or no was the minimal answer. She probed more and more and more, and I just wasn't up for it. Finally, I said, "I really don't want to talk about this. Things are fine. I just don't want to talk about it."

RM: A reasonable request.

N: Well, she just could not let it go. She came back and really wanted to be reassured so much. I just didn't have the energy. I don't have the psychic energy to go back through the stages of development that have gotten us here—that's number one. Number two, the last two months or so have been a different process. It hasn't been an imagery process. It's been a much more explicitly spiritual process that I couldn't unpack on the telephone. I just could not revisit all of that and explain it. The fundamental stuff of Christianity is not what works for her.

RM: You are in a different zone now.

N: Yes, thank you, that's good. It is different for me. Again, I had to say I really don't want to talk about it—it's too hard. That night, Al helped me write her an email. I said I appreciated everything she had done. I could never have gotten to where I am without the work we've done in the past two years, and I'm not in any way denigrating the process or its outcome. I was just moving past there, and I can't fully articulate it.

Commentary: *The tension Nell feels with Mary is similar to her response when Kristin barged into her room, asked for a hug, and tickled her feet. Like the physical boundary violation of Kristin, Mary's need for affirmation of her guided-imagery intervention is an intrusion on Nell's world, a psychological boundary violation. Good therapists manage to separate their own needs from those of the patient. Mary's dual relationship with Nell as friend and therapist complicates their dynamic, and ultimately, Nell rejects the therapist to reclaim her friend.*

RM: You have always spoken with deep affection for Mary and your work with her.

N: The last time we had gone through a round of "Please, could you back off?" she had nursed it for a couple of weeks as a repudiation of her methods and her guided-imagery work. I realized that she very much needed validation for herself. She was not secure. This time, she sent a card by overnight mail. I want you to read that. I love that card.

RM: The card has this printed message, "We give comfort and receive comfort sometimes at the same time," and then Mary's written words (Box 9.1).

Box 9.1 Mary's words, mailed to Nell in a card

Dear Nellie,

I received your email this morning and was so grateful as it helped me understand just where you are and to accept that with gratitude. I realize that your momentum is forward and letting go is a violent part of that process that orients the ways we have communicated in the past. Very sadly I realized also I cannot walk with you on your path in all the ways we have in the past and I know I'm not meant to, especially now. I love you dearly, Nell. I deeply respect your life and how you are living it now. I trust you are held. I thank you for being a superb friend to me and a role model on such a challenging journey. If our paths cross in the rain or within a sun or moonbeam it will be in love always.

Mary

N: Isn't that beautiful? Isn't that wonderful?

RM: "If our paths cross in the rain or within a sun or moonbeam, it will be in love always." That is beautiful.

N: She sent it by overnight mail. Mary doesn't like to wait for things! (Laughs.)

RM: The moon is full, and when the moon is full—

N: The moon is my reminder—we are on schedule. Remember, the moon is my metronome.

RM: Yes, I remember. The moon is your guide and your anchor.

N: It marks the time. Remember in my vision?

RM: Oh, yes. I remember your vision of peacefulness assured by a guiding light, the light of the moon, right outside your window.

N: The moon is my guide, in that sense. The moon can say if I am on schedule. But it really is an organic process. There is nothing inherently alarming about what's going on. All is as it is supposed to be.

RM: I agree with the moon. There is a peacefulness about your home that stays with me as I leave.

N: Thank you. Now, I am ready for a poem.

RM: Before I read, can you tell me how you're doing with the pain management, with morphine?

N: I am sleeping. When I need morphine, it works. I think that the acupuncture helped a lot, too. It really knocked out some cramping around the ribs, the area that is very stressed.

RM: It was a good idea to get your acupuncture person to do a home session.

N: It was a desperate act because I was in so much pain all the time. It was a very, very specific area. She identified it as following a particular rib from front to back. The rib right over where the liver is. She worked on it for quite a while with the tuning forks. It is much better. It doesn't flare up.

RM: Good. OK, I have two poems, both by Ted Kooser. He is the Pulitzer Prize–winning author of *Delights and Shadows*. He wrote "Skater," which I gave you.[3]

N: Yes, I remember—to help me with fear—ice skating in the dark.

RM: The first poem is "Surviving" (Box 9.2) and the second one is "The Early Bird."

N: Very observant—such detail.

RM: Kooser was treated for tongue cancer in 1998. I sent him the article, "Turning Toward Death Together: Conversation in Mortal Time," by Michael Cowan and me; he wrote out a gracious response via postcard, the same medium he used to create his book, *Winter Morning Walks: One Hundred Postcards to Jim Harrison*. It's poetry about his diagnosis and treatment of cancer.

N: Oh my!

RM: I saw him on a webcast where he was interviewing John Prine at the Library of Congress.[4] He talked about his cancer, and they started discussing their experience of cancer. Ted Kooser has been through the wringer. He has been acquainted with mortal

---

Box 9.2   Surviving

Ted Kooser

> There are days when the fear of death
> Is as unambiguous as light. It illuminates
> Everything. Without it, I might not
> Have noticed this ladybird beetle,
> Bright as a drop of blood
> On the window's white sill.
> Her head no bigger than a period,
> Her eyes like needle points,
> She has stopped for a moment to rest,
> Knees locked, wing covers hiding
> The delicate lace of her wings.
> As the fear of death, so attentive
> To everything living, comes near her,
> The tiny antennae stop moving.

---

time. When I read this next poem, I thought of you in relation to bird watching. It's called "The Early Bird." (Box 9.3).

N: Perfect.

RM: "Hauling the heavy / bucket of dawn / up from the darkness, / note over note / and letting us drink." What a promise!

N: Perfect poem. That is a perfect poem.

RM: Tomorrow, as you're rousing early in the morning, noon, or night, perhaps you'll hear an early bird, hauling the heavy bucket of dawn up.

N: That's lovely. Thank you.

Final Commentary: Kooser's elegant poem "Surviving" reflects the comforting idea that the prospect of death can be illuminating. Indeed, Nell's regular reflections about living and dying are the illuminating source of our conversation. However, the content of our talks does not hover over death relentlessly. Staying too close to the prospect of our own ending can be depressing and emotionally draining. The poem "The Early Bird" is a refreshing reminder of the birds that give life to Nell each day as they chatter away at the feeders. The idea that dawn can be hauled up from the darkness speaks to the notion that perhaps life can be found even in the darkness of death. In our next dialogue, Nell finds new life through a simple medical procedure that exacted a toll on her.

Box 9.3 The Early Bird

Ted Kooser

Still dark, and raining hard
on a cold May morning

and yet the early bird
is out there chirping,

chirping its sweet-sour
wooden-pulley notes,

pleased, it would seem,
to be given work,

hauling the heavy
bucket of dawn

up from the darkness,
note over note
and letting us drink.

Notes

1. Shades of Praise is an interracial gospel choir from New Orleans. It was co-founded by Michael Cowan, my co-author of *The art of conversation through serious illness: Lessons for caregivers* (2010; New York: Oxford University Press). See https://www.shadesofpraise.org/.

2. Ricoeur, P. (2009). *Living up to death* (p. 17). Chicago: University of Chicago Press.

3. Kooser, T. (2004). *Delights and shadows* (pp. 75, 81). Port Townsend, WA: Copper Canyon Press. In Chapter 5, Nell compared her situation to a person ice skating in the dark. I subsequently gave her the poem "The Skater" (p. 17).

4. "A literary evening with John Prine and Ted Kooser" was held in Coolidge Auditorium on March 9, 2005, during Kooser's first term as U.S. Poet Laureate. The webcast is one of the Library's most popular. https://www. loc.gov/item/webcast-3677/

10

May 30, 2005—Far from Home

When it's over, I want to say: all my life
I was a bride married to amazement.

> Oliver, M. (1992). *New and selected poems* (p. 10).
> Boston: Beacon Press.

Main Themes: Leaving the safety of home, experiencing emotional vulnerability and anxiety at the hospital, and seeking spiritual sustenance.

Nell requested a transfusion for profound lack of energy due to her low hemoglobin. During the 10-hour odyssey to the hospital, she met helpful healthcare providers and saw many opportunities to express her gratitude. Al and Anna accompanied her and helped ease her distress. Nevertheless, anxiety spiked badly when she discovered that her do-not-resuscitate (DNR) form was still at home, hanging prominently on the wall above her bed. Nell recognized that resuscitation success rates are only about 30 percent for people over 65 and that her tumor will continue to grow, eventually closing off life; in any case, she does not want to be kept alive artificially. Fortunately, Anna later brought the DNR to the hospital. It acts as a security object for Nell, like the rosary she frequently holds.

Nell speaks of finding refuge and strength in scripture, especially Psalm 139. We begin the meeting with Nell describing her ambulance and hospital adventure, made tolerable by her curiosity.

Dialogue 10

N: This 10-hour marathon to get a transfusion is the first time I've been out of Creekside Apartments since the 23rd of February! I had an infantile reaction when I left my DNR behind. The DNR document is in the category with holding on to the rosary—not saying it, but having it in my hand. There is something steadying about the familiarity of being at home, too, and I did not realize that was at work. This place against which I have rebelled so thoroughly has become my safe place. I was really reluctant not to be here.

RM: You feel safe here, and a 10-hour marathon away was no picnic. What a hard scene!

N: Yes! I think it has to do with the simple feeling of elementary control. There is really no control, but it feels as if we've woven a safety net into this room and this apartment. It is custom-tailored for all the little problems, like where the fan tripod is, so I don't fall over it. Just every little thing that I have learned for safety and reassurance. In the hospital, I was in a room without a window, and by the end of the day, I became claustrophobic.

RM: It sounds like a very hard, tiring trip.

N: This claustrophobia has never happened before. Talking to you about it now helps me clarify. One of my reactions then was to have a pathetic emotionality. I mean, all these 30-year-old nurses are calling me baby, honey, and sweetie. (Laughs.) They are saying, "You poor baby." They were overwhelmed by how tiny and frail I am. I felt like a baby, and I was thanking everybody all the time—the least little thing. I just was in a wash of emotions triggered by disorientation. I found that fascinating. This is my question for your feedback: What are the reasons for the emotions and the disequilibrium? Was I so on the edge and don't have reserves of emotions and stability, at all?! I do fundamentally, but day to day, I depend very much on my environment and have a routine. I was just simply astonished at how quickly that can go away.

RM: How quickly reserves and your sense of emotional equilibrium can go away?

N: Yes. The reserves get drawn down. The equilibrium is gone. I was astonished by that.

RM: Well, you just said a lot, especially the change of environment from this cocoon of warmth and security. It reminds me of Lynn Felder's poem "Cocooning," which we read.[1] You left your cocoon here. The change of environment, the physical demands of traveling from this room to the ambulance and from the ambulance to the hospital, and I imagine you changed beds and then changed to a wheelchair on arrival?

N: A gurney.

RM: OK, so you had a lot of physical movement and change. Maybe even discomfort?

N: Yes.

RM: The transfusion procedure itself can feel invasive. I'm getting the picture of many people you encountered requiring a lot of communication energy from you. And an unusual kind of energy coming your way that is not what you are accustomed to—being called *honey*, *sweetie*. I didn't hear a completely negative reaction to that—more like curiosity. It wasn't necessarily negative or positive?

N: Yes. It was surprising.

RM: Surprising?

N: You know me very well, and you know the decades of practice at being competent that make me up.

RM: Yes, I do good doctor. (Chuckles.)

N: (Chuckles.) That's who I am. Now I find myself appropriately at the mercy of others, literally. I am a baby in practical, functional terms, and I did not resist. A man and a woman, Stan and Agnes, staffed the ambulance. Stan was driving, and Agnes was in the back—muscular, sort of Slavic build. She was wearing this bracelet, and she wanted to give it to me. Normally, I would say, "Oh, no, no, you keep it." But I could see that she really wanted me to have it; it meant a lot to her to give it to me. She gave it to me, and it went up to my shoulder. (Laughs.) She still wanted me to have it, so I kept it on for the return trip and then took it off. Well, it's just more stuff, but I could feel her reaching out and the desire to be helpful. She wanted to do more than just set me on the gurney and stuff me in the ambulance. It was very generous, very kind.

RM: So you had kindness and generosity coming your way, and it felt different. You are a very competent adult. The message was not that you are incompetent but that you are now a person who could be called *baby, sweetie*, not the kind of name you normally evoke. For lots of reasons, it's not your style to encourage being treated in a *sweetie, there-there* sort of way.

N: Yes, yes.

Commentary: *Nell is a curious participant in, and observer of, the reactions of her caregivers throughout her hospital visit. Her view of herself as a competent adult is challenged; even though she is not treated poorly, being called* honey *and* baby *feels patronizing and infantilizing. Her attendants mean no harm, hardly noticing that they are speaking to her as they might to a child. Agnes doesn't notice that her generous gift of an ill-fitting bracelet is embarrassing.*

This experience is new to Nell. She is seeing herself through the eyes of her professional caregivers and recognizes how her changed body reflects a changed identity. The use of terms challenging her adult identity would normally set her on edge, yet she finds it both comforting and fascinating, a curious diversion. Curiosity in a new situation can reduce stress, but her reactions may also provide a measure of how her physical decline is paralleled by psychological changes. She accepts her new status as a person who has less control over her body and her fate. She is letting go of her self in this world.

RM: I also hear the comfort of holding the rosary or other security items was missing. You didn't have anything to hold on to physically.

N: I didn't have Amber, and I realized this is tactile. It was about tactility, if there is such a word, and the comfort of holding something. I have found lately that Amber often is just here. If I'm not touching Amber, he will stretch out his arm and lean on me. He seems to need that as much as I do. I know that there have been studies that confirm this. I find myself just stroking him. It is very comforting. It's relaxing. It reduces that kind of background tension that is there with the difficulty of being awake or the difficulty of getting to sleep.

RM: So Amber was gone; the rosary was gone; your usual orienting surroundings were gone. How about Al? Was Al there?

N: Al was there, and Anna, bless her heart—she came for the entire ordeal. I had forgotten to pack up my DNR, and when I got to the hospital, I panicked because it was not clear to them immediately that it was on file. It should be the top line. It should be right there with your insurance number, in the system, uniformly, everywhere—it should be! I was afraid of something happening, so I wouldn't let myself nap. Finally, Anna said, "Would you like to take a nap?" I said I would love to take a nap, but I can't because I forgot the DNR form! She went back to our apartment and got my DNR off the wall.

RM: Bless her. I can just see you in a half-awake sleep state, somebody about to clamp down on you, and you come out with, "Don't you dare keep me alive!"

N: Yes, you bet. (Laughs.)

RM: "I will kill you if you try to keep me alive!"

N: That's right! (Laughs.)

RM: But you're not murderous. That wouldn't be you. (Laughs.)

N: "I'll just die if you try to keep me alive!" (Laughs.)

Commentary: One of Nell's most enduring qualities is her sense of humor, even during the most difficult times. In this instance, she is able to chuckle at the possibility of arguing with someone who might attempt to use extraordinary means to keep her alive. She wants to give over to her own death, to leave the world without being yoked to tubes and machines. These light moments lighten our serious conversation about mortality. Hovering over the facts of death too long can spark intense anxiety.

RM: I think I understand the picture; you painted it very clearly. Was it worth it?

N: Yes. I came back home after the transfusion, and I had a burst of energy. I immediately cleaned the litter box. Amber was so distraught at having been left alone all day. I tidied up all his stuff and reassured him. I made sandwiches and promptly then was much too tired to eat, so I made myself a milkshake and soon thereafter went to bed. I had another of those feelings: I have turned the corner—something has changed definitively. It was a sinking feeling. And I had almost a mythical feeling about borrowing someone else's blood to keep me alive.

RM: Sinking?

Commentary: Nell can move quickly from laughter to deep sadness. She names a sinking feeling and recognizes that her downward spiral is approaching the ending she both welcomes and fears. It's the finality, the acceptance of nonbeing, and the "end of me" that can sink a heart. She wisely reached for the presence and love of Al for comfort.

N: Yes, there is a kind of finality to it. I asked Al to come in and read this psalm to me that I love, Psalm 139. We sang it as a hymn. "Lord, you have searched me and known me; you know my goings out and my comings." I asked him to pray with me. In 21 years of marriage, I've never asked either of those things. It was a very rich and strengthening moment.

RM: You are sharing very special moments with Al and others.

N: Yes. I called Lori and asked her to bring me a missalette and hymnal, so I can have more food for my spirit. Right now, I'm just jumping around amongst what I am familiar with in scripture, but I need some more structure. I just want you to think with me about meditation in this time. I don't know if there are resources that you know of already. The goal is to have a four-legged stool to nurture my spirituality.[2] I need to make it more structured and reliable. Maybe somebody has talked with you before about this?

RM: Yes. You're thinking of scripture and/or poetry, mainly scripture?

N: Scripture, prayers, and poetry.

RM: Anthony de Mello comes to mind.[3] He is an Indian Jesuit priest and psychotherapist. He has a book of writings. I like your idea with regard to structure. Having a daily reflective prayer time with Al, Lori, Fr. Bob, or whoever would want to read scripture or some words that speak to you. I have a poem by Mary Oliver you may like. It's called "When Death Comes."[4] I would like to read it to you.

N: Yes, please do (Box 10.1).

N: Oh! That is so wonderful. It's beautiful.

Commentary: *This poem (Box 10.1) speaks to Nell as she is welcoming death's arrival. She will not "end up simply having visited this world." She indeed is a "bride married to amazement"—the amazement of the world around her, Creekside Apartments, the cardinals that greet her in the morning, the storm clouds that rumble across her landscape, the bright moon that serves as her guide and anchor.*

RM: Married to amazement. There's amazement right here, with you and Al.

N: That's true. Now, I have one for you to read aloud. This is Donald Justice. Do you know Donald Justice?[5]

Box 10.1 When Death Comes

Mary Oliver

When death comes
like the hungry bear in autumn;
when death comes and takes all the bright coins from
   his purse
to buy me, and snaps the purse shut;
when death comes
like the measles-pox;
when death comes
like an iceberg between the shoulder blades,
I want to step through the door full of curiosity, wondering:
what is it going to be like, that cottage of darkness?
And therefore I look upon everything
as a brotherhood and a sisterhood,
and I look upon time as no more than an idea,
and I consider eternity as another possibility,
and I think of each life as a flower, as common
as a field daisy, and as singular,
and each name a comfortable music in the mouth
ascending as all music does, toward silence,
and each body a lion of courage, and something
precious to the earth.
When it's over, I want to say: all my life
I was a bride married to amazement.

RM: No (see Box 10.2).

N: Isn't that lovely?

RM: Yes. How did you happen to come upon this, now?

N: One day when I was very weak and physically low, Anna was
visiting. She is very tender-hearted. She just quoted the whole

thing from memory. She was holding my hand, and she just came forth with that poem. I asked her to give me a copy of it. I was thinking of looking for it online and making you a copy.

RM: Thank you. It is a beautiful poem.

Box 10.2 There Is a Gold Light in Certain Old Paintings

Donald Justice

1

There is a gold light in certain old paintings
That represents a diffusion of sunlight.
It is like happiness, when we are happy.
It comes from everywhere and nowhere at once, this light,
And the poor soldiers sprawled at the foot of the cross
Share in its charity equally with the cross.

2

Orpheus hesitated beside the black river.
With so much to look forward to he looked back.
We think he sang then, but the song is lost.
At least he had seen once more the beloved back.
I say the song went this way: *O prolong*
Now the sorrow if that is all there is to prolong.

3

The world is very dusty, uncle. Let us work.
One day the sickness shall pass from the earth for good.
The orchard will bloom; someone will play the guitar.
Our work will be seen as strong and clean and good.
And all that we suffered through having existed
Shall be forgotten as though it had never existed.

Commentary: *Nell loves this poem by Donald Justice because it is a meditation on art and mythology as they relate to daily life. Nell has a PhD in art history. She appreciates the poem within the religious context and the notion that the same sun will shine on all of us, regardless of religious inclination. The idea that sickness will pass and all suffering be forgotten at our death comforts Nell.*

N: Now, a prayer would be nice. Can you put your hand here on my abdomen and pray with me?

RM: Yes, I can. And Al will join the circle here.

AL: Certainly.

RM: Lord, we thank you for this time, for the light that shines within and around Nell and Al here in this home, full of grace, this cocoon of love and caring. This is a safe place, a home that will always be an oasis in this world, a place of peace. We ask for gratitude for each day, for everything at our table, even if it is not what we ordered. We thank you for the gift of life and especially the light and the moon that anchors, guides, and beckons Nell. Amen.

N AND AL: Thank you so much.

RM: Sleep well. No dancing tonight.

AL: No dancing tonight.

RM: Maybe a little bit of French Open or something on TV? Maybe you will be up and about?

N: Yes, I have a new wheelchair, so I can move about.

RM: No speeding, all right?

N: (Laughs.) Thank you, Dick.

Final Commentary: *I am honored that Nell asks me to pray, as I know it is important to her and brings the three of us together in a healing circle. While I am not trained in pastoral counseling, I am comfortable with spiritual discussion, prayer, and questions regarding ultimate meaning, which for me include reaching for mystery,* the transcendent, and the force that connects all inhabitants of our universe.

When we ended with a prayer tonight, imagery and thoughts of the moon were prominent. It is in the last quarter, about 50 percent visible. The moon represents powerful feminine energy. It signifies wisdom, intuition, birth, death, reincarnation, and a spiritual connection. It is an anchor and a beacon for Nell. It connects her to the world and beckons her to the heavens.

Ending the session with poetry and prayer creates a moment that joins Nell, Al, and me. We have gotten closer over these weeks, meeting in their home, and Al has begun to participate more actively. He is a private, reserved man but now, more than ever, responsive to Nell's emotional needs. I am glad to see that he feels comfortable joining us and expressing his care for Nell. At this very special time in their marriage, the prospect of death has brought them closer together. Nell has a physical and emotional place of safety and a home to launch from—a comforting realization. It is a welcome refuge from the grief of loss that emerges in our next dialogue.

Notes

1. See Box 8.1 in Chapter 8.
2. Thomas Hübl, a spiritual teacher, uses the metaphor of the stable four-legged stool to encapsulate a framework for inspiration and resilience. See Ward, N. (2018, December 10). A four-legged stool. *Education Connected.* https://educationconnected.co.uk/general-news/a-four-legged-stool/
3. De Mello, A. (1984). *The song of the bird.* New York: Doubleday.
4. Oliver, M. (1992). *New and selected poems* (pp. 10–11). Boston: Beacon Press.
5. Justice, D. (2004). There is a gold light in certain old paintings. In *Collected poems.* New York: Knopf. https://www.poeticous.com/donald-justice/there-is-a-gold-light-in-certain-old-paintings?al=t&laf=t&lns=j&locale=fr/

11

June 7, 2005—Grief and Sadness

Give sorrow words: the grief that does not speak
Whispers the o'er-fraught heart and bids it break.
Shakespeare, *Macbeth*, Act 4, Scene 3, ll. 209–210

Main Themes: Grief, loss, and sadness; Nell's awareness that she is losing 20 years of expected lifespan; finding consolation in Buddhism and faith in a God who helps her accept fate.

Nell's tumor is growing noticeably; her abdomen is grossly distended. I have not seen her for eight days, a long time at this point in her disease trajectory. Tonight she looks weary, yet her conversational energy is strong and her spirits are high. Hospice has provided a hospital bed, which allows her to get up and down more easily. Her legs are swollen, and her walking is limited. She eats very little. Nonetheless, she continues to live well as she approaches death, and our dialogue reflects experiences of both mourning and cheer. Nell has read and edited the transcript of our earlier dialogue and begins our conversation humorously.

Dialogue 11

N: In our May 17 discussion, there is a corner being turned after I had beaten that horse into the ground about the timing of my death. (Laughs.) The theme on the 17th was discovering that

I was happy and realizing that it was all right to be happy and alive! It's not betraying my mission if I do not die on schedule or conform to a median life expectancy.

RM: Yes, it is OK to be alive and even happy!

Commentary: Nell finds humor in what seems like a paradox: Is it possible to be both open to death's approach and happy to be alive? Sadness and cheerfulness are threaded throughout our conversations. Nell has become accustomed to their pairing but finds it unsatisfying. She appears restless with unexpressed sadness. At times, she has questioned her lack of grief at her loss. All that is about to change.

N: I think it is worth putting down on paper what I'd like to salvage. The ideas from our conversation about death on May 17 are very important to me. The way Buber and Roethke frame it is so nicely because it really comes to the same thing as prayer in a way.[1] Letting go of the structure of expectations. In the Buber piece, expectations in relationships and expectations of the structure and function of mysticism. In Roethke, it's about nature.[2] Both of them come down to listening, being observant, being open, and being fully present in the moment. I think being present in the moment is some form of transcendence, and that is the puzzle, the paradox. It gives one permission to be happy and alive in the moment and just to say thank you, which is where I am headed—gratitude.

RM: Yes, Nell, your gratitude shines always.

N: I have been revisiting this book on contemplative prayer. In a few periods in my life, I was into contemplative prayer. I don't know if we talked about this much.

RM: We haven't, no.

N: I'm very eager to have that kind of openness, presence, and total availability to the present. What I'm talking about is a resource in every religion. It's just that I'm learning it in our religion. I don't want our dialogues to become Christianized to the exclusion of a Buddhist perspective or a Jewish perspective, but it's time for the faith dimension to be unabashedly there because that's what's happening for me.

RM: Well, I do not experience your reflections as being narrow or sectarian. They are grounded in Christianity but very broad in reach in so many ways, including poetry and your reflections.

N: Can closure come from this approach?

RM: Yes. Buddhist, Jewish, Protestant, Christian, Hindu—all have their own rituals around death. I'm not a religious scholar, so I am not very familiar with rituals in each. You have the idea of being grounded in your faith and open to many others. I am reminded of this as I see the statue of the Buddha on your shelf. I was at the Sackler Gallery in Washington yesterday, and there I met images of the Buddha and a bodhisattva by the name of Guanyin, the bodhisattva of compassion. I thought of you.

N: You are a bodhisattva.[3] It's very true.

RM: That is very kind of you to say now and a while back. It is very generous to me, as I now have a better idea of what it means to be a bodhisattva. I learned that in Buddhist philosophy, a bodhisattva is one that helps usher others into nirvana—not entering there with them, but as a guide for the journey. Guanyin happens to start out male and then evolves into a higher form of being, female, transcending gender. It's a wonderful way to symbolize this idea of compassion. I thought of you and your use of the word *bodhisattva* in relation to me. It's a special compliment.

N: Yes, evolving into a higher form—female! (Laughs.) I think what Buddhism offers, besides the notion of nonbeing as a way of life, is compassion as the way to connect with the world and as a way to be responsible to the world, whereas Christianity has creeds and liturgies and rules. A book that I'm almost ready to pass on to you is on the second shelf from the bottom. It has a red spine and a gold front. It's called *The Tibetan Book of Living and Dying.*[4] Do you know this book?

RM: I've heard of *The Tibetan Book of the Dead*.

N: This book is different. It has a very good exposition of *tonglen* as practiced—of participating in the suffering of others.[5] Tonglen is a core concept of Buddhism. It has been popularized to some extent. The whole notion of relating to the suffering of someone else by entering into it with them is the heart of tonglen, and it's the heart of what a bodhisattva does. A bodhisattva is a person who has attained enlightenment and is qualified to pass over and elects to stay on this side of enlightenment for the sake of ushering other people along the way. It is a gift in the way it is given. The heart of Buddhism has an enormous amount to offer us. We Christians have often gotten stuck in personal salvation and personal benefit. This is a more generous approach.

RM: I agree, although I am a long way from enlightenment. You sound like a Buddhist Catholic speaking!

N: (Laughs.) Yes, I suppose I am becoming a hybrid! I'm not going to read it again because I don't have the time or the strength. I didn't want to lay a bunch of Buddhist concepts on you, but these are very useful ideas. For example, this notion of *bardo*, a special space. I don't truly understand it. It's the space of passing over into death and whatever comes next.

RM: Bardo?

N: There is a chapter in the book on the concept of bardo—the state of existence between death and rebirth. You really need to have this book, if you don't mind? I don't want to impose my library on you.

RM: Of course, thank you. It's a wonderful gift. I first heard the name Rinpoche in the writings of Ken Wilbur, a book called *Grace and Grit*. It is both a scholarly work and a personal story of his journey with wife Treya, as she was being treated for breast cancer.[6] Wilbur is a brilliant thinker. He draws upon Buddhist concepts, philosophy, throughout the book. He made the medical, mystical journey toward death with Treya. But the book you have is not the same as *The Tibetan Book of the Dead*?

N: No, it's a reflection on *The Tibetan Book of the Dead*. I am revisiting it now and inclined to pass it on to you, as it is a teaching. *Rinpoche* is just a word for teacher. In the book, a woman gets deeply into Buddhism. Her master assigns her to teach *The Book of the Dead* for summer school at the Buddhist Center in Colorado. She undertakes it as a splendid manual on being present for other people's dying, their pain and suffering, and for pain and suffering in life in general. In each section, she identifies a theme with meditation ideas for the theme and practical applications for the themes. She is extremely good about helping practitioners get the *self* out of the way and always being present.

RM: Getting your *self* out of the way, yes!

N: This book is coming to you. I'm just cherishing it for a while. I told you about it a long time ago. I just need to be regrounded in it before passing it on. You have work to do with this book.

RM: OK. Now, what did you think of these books by Fredrick Buechner[7] and Anthony de Mello?[8]

N: Well, I enjoyed them very much. I've spent more time with Buechner. The one by de Mello—I haven't had much reading time.

RM: de Mello has short writings. He gives you something to chew on. It's practical wisdom.

N: Yes, and good and true. Al and I have a little ritual at night now where we do the readings for a day, and then we pray together, and then we switch, and Al reads something light until I'm dozing and ready to go to sleep.

RM: He talks you to sleep. That's wonderful.

N: Yes, it is very, very nice. That's developing, and it's good for both of us, I think. We need to connect, you know. And Al needs the time.

RM: Yes, you are connecting with Al. Does Lori come out as well?

N: Lori came yesterday. Fr. Bob came Sunday. I'm being pelted with kindness. (Laughs.)

RM: You're getting a good spiritual talking-to, aren't you? (Laughter.)

N: Yes. That's right! Yep.

RM: You are coming together in prayer. Is Al doing OK with it?

N: Yes, he is OK with prayer. Al was struck the other night by the readings around suffering. It gave him a place to acknowledge that we are suffering and to use the word *suffering*. I think that is what it does for him—gives him words for our suffering. Otherwise, he has to be strong.

RM: Well, that's a good opening because he sure does lead with his strength. I can feel it, and yet I know there is a lot more there.

N: Yes, there is, and now we are sharing it.

RM: Excellent.

Commentary: At times, Nell has felt emotionally distant from Al, and she feared this feeling would increase following his diagnosis of Alzheimer's disease. However, her illness has ushered in a new form of intimacy between them, revolving around shared time in their apartment. Even as death approaches, Nell is finding possibilities in their relationship as a source of comfort and sadness. Now she has more to lose.

N: Did you get my big email?

RM: No, I haven't been into email.

N: I did a big email yesterday to encourage and reward people who have refrained from telephoning because I just thought I need to "lock the gate," as they say. Don't call. But there needs to be more reciprocity in it. I told everybody what was going on here and talked about Al. I think you will appreciate it. I'll try to do that periodically because people tend to be sweet, sending cards and notes and pictures and stuff, and I can't answer everybody. I am grateful for them, keeping them in my prayers. I made essentially a kind of stay-in-touch list in the address book and sent it to everybody. What do you think? (Box 11.1).

Box 11.1 Nell's "letting go" email to friends

Dear Loved Ones,

Over the past few weeks, because I have become so weak and must struggle to hear and talk on the phone, I have been asking each of you to forego telephoning and to use e-mail or snail mail instead. Everyone has been wonderful. In lieu of phone calls, you send photos and poems and descriptions of your families' goings-on, and of the weather and your thoughts in general. I check e-mail with real pleasure, although sometimes many days pass before I can answer. Thank you, for understanding and adapting.

Let me tell you about things that are going on here. For some of you, this is no-news; for others it is the first time I've had a chance to write you. So please bear with. On the health side, I have been really helped by hospice services, including a trans-fusion, which I received a week ago last Saturday. My hemo-globin had gotten low. I had to go to the hospital by ambulance for the procedure and it took all day, but it was well worth the effort in the gift of energy. Oxygen continues to be most helpful, as has the introduction of a real hospital bed and a real wheel-chair. The wheelchair lets me have some time out of bed, which means Al and I can often sit up together for ritual TV watching. We're putting Netflix through its paces, and WE WOULD LOVE to hear about movies you especially recommend. We always end the day by reading together (Al reads to me) and listening to music. Al and I are glad for this time together.

We are grateful for faithful friends—especially Anna, Pat, and Bill—who bring groceries, administer back rubs, and generally brighten our days. Just today, for example, Anna brought the first blueberries of the season—such a treat—as she had earlier brought the first strawberries, and her own inimitable strawberry jam. Pat puts her massage skills, learned in Girl Scouts, to much appreciated good use. And Bill does mechanical-genius things, like installing a touch-activated reading light within reach of the bed, and taking Al on essential errands.

We have also been gifted by the ministry of friends and staff at church. Lori brings communion weekly, and both Brother Jay and Fr. Bob have administered the anointing of the sick. Dr. Richard McQuellon, who directs the Psychosocial Oncology & Cancer Patient Support programs at the Comprehensive Cancer Center of Baptist Hospital, has been a wonderful counselor and guide as I've tried to navigate this journey to death. He and I are now sharing a reflective writing/dialogue process. He plans to use these papers in his practice and as he continues to develop his concept of "mortal time."

Al remains the Rock, the quiet, most graceful friend I've ever been graced to know. Still, I am sure the price is high for him, and I solicit your prayers for his peace and well-being.

Many of you are praying for both of us. We feel and know your support. In turn we pray for your happiness and safe-keeping. Thank you for being our friends. And thank you again for your courtesy regarding the phone.

With love, Nell

RM: That is a fine idea, allowing yourself the possibility of wishing all well and praying for everyone who has touched you, keeping them in your heart, not necessarily emailing.

N: Yep, that's the idea.

Commentary: Nell's "letting-go" email to friends was a big step for her.

RM: You do this already—keeping your dear ones in your heart. You are full of gratitude.

N: I feel it. The psalm yesterday was Psalm 34, referenced in the lectionary, a list of scriptural readings for the day. I looked up the whole version, and I got the pith of it and left out a lot of talk. Look at this. I wrote to my cousin John; he said it's paradoxical, but it's true.

> I will bless the Lord at all times for his praise. It shall be ever in my mouth.
> Let my soul glory in the Lord. And lo you will hear me and be glad.
> Glorify the Lord with me, let us extol His name!
> I sought the Lord, and he answered me and delivered me from all my fears. Look to him and be radiant with joy and your faces may not blush with shame. And the poor one called out. The Lord heard and from all his distress, he saved him. The angel of the Lord encamps around those who fear and delivers them. Taste and see how good the Lord is! Bless the person who takes refuge in him!

RM: This reading touched you. You and Al read something like this each day?

N: At night. It's how we end the day. Then I put on the Theresa Schroeder-Sheker CD *Rosa Mystica* and turn the light off. Al sits here for 10 to 15 minutes and then goes to his room. I leave *Rosa Mystica* on until it finishes, so we fall asleep to the same music. It's very nice. That CD has gotten more wear. I hope you did thank her in some way.

RM: Yes, I did. I will email to thank her again. Her heroic efforts got the CD to us quickly!

N: That's good. It is fantastic. And, I've done all the talking I can do. It's your turn.

RM: You may have to do a little bit more because I have some inquiries. When we talked on the phone Friday, you had had an exchange with Sally that was very upsetting. I want to come back to that and see how it settled for you.

N: I think you calmed me right away by reminding me of our foundation. I was off my pins. I wasn't on foundation. I know I was so tired. It was a good warning to me that the old body/mind is still interacting. Step one was just getting back on my foundation and remembering the kind of spirituality that Sally has is very unique, with traps in it. Mostly, it makes you guilty. Somehow, after our talk, it was like turning on a dime. It was OK. I did the things you reminded me to do—the breathing, the quiet recollection, the *Rosa Mystica* music, holding on to the rosary, just being still—and I felt much stronger. I haven't had an attack like that again. But it was upsetting. I was just very vulnerable right then. Funny, it's not like I've had any epiphanies since then, but I just feel more steady. I think it's the reading–prayer connection that provides a theme.

Commentary: *Nell's professional caregiver Sally has a unique spirituality and religious view that is very different from Nell's. While Sally had good intentions, her efforts to convert Nell to her way of thinking about God were upsetting. Nell is too weak and vulnerable to explain her version of Christianity, which has become more important as she nears the end. She is seeking her own spiritual path now and cannot tolerate the intrusion of an imposed fundamental religious framework. This particular interaction was intrusive and triggered intense rumination and agitation.*

I am listening for the areas cancer patients must manage: disease and symptom management, interpersonal relationships, distressing thoughts and feelings and the role changes and practical demands of the day. Nell's relationship with Sally is crucial. Sally helps with daily activities. She is a close companion with access to Nell's heart. Nell depends on her. Now, two of these areas of coping in cancer care have been disrupted: the conflicted interpersonal relationship and the cascade of thoughts and feelings it stirred up.

RM: You are steadying yourself with prayer, with a ritual, Al, music, with remembering *your* path, not Sally's. Yet you have always been open to others.

N: Well, more than I realize, I think. I still haven't recognized sorrow in myself. I think that is part of where my weakness was and probably is. Sorrow—because I am young, and I probably would not have reason to know that story well—the story of Jephthah's daughter in the Bible—without this illness, this breast cancer.

RM: The story of Jephthah?

N: Jephthah is a judge who offers his daughter as a burnt sacrifice to the Lord, and she assents. He's made this pledge to God that if he wins the big battle, he will sacrifice whoever comes out of his house to greet him when he returns home. Who comes first? His daughter, who has come out to greet him. He says, "Oh, no, you've ruined my life because now I have to kill you!" His daughter says, "It's all right. If you made a promise to God, then that's what you have to do. Give me three weeks to go into the hills with my women friends and mourn my virginity."

RM: This story tugs at your heart. I can see tears in your eyes.

N: Please take my hand. I think that in all the turmoil of doing and managing and preparing, I haven't left room to be sad. When I ran out of strength that day talking with Sally, I just was completely out of energy. I think that is where my sadness inserted itself.

RM: You were upset and sad as well. Were you able to feel your sadness?

N: Not right away but soon thereafter. Then I had this impish thought that I would like the TV to come; I would like a few weeks with the television like Jephthah's daughter and the maidens in the mountains (chuckles). That would be my celebration, so then my sense of humor returned. Can you put your hand back on mine? It is so nice.

RM: Yes, sure.

N: Thank you. But is that all I can say on that? I need to acknowledge that I regret not having the next 20 years.

RM: Yes, of course. I regret it, too, and appreciate your words and your willingness to open your heart to what is there, whether it be joy or the sadness. Your heart is so well attuned. Now you are sad.

N: Thank you. (Tears; long pause.)

Commentary: Nell is more comfortable with rational analysis than expressing her sadness and emotional intensity. However, she recognizes her deep sadness and this evening sheds tears, which she has done on occasion as she grieves the loss of her good life. She is not one to stay stuck in sadness or grieving. She appreciates irony even at the end. My task is to help her navigate her path, which includes sadness, grieving, and humor along the way.

RM: I heard you say Sally was misinterpreting your experience, which knocked you off your pins, knocked you off your foundation. What I didn't hear on the phone but hear in your voice today is more sadness, not fear. Now you are naming your sadness more clearly. It's not required to have long, deep grieving periods. It is not your way to remain in sadness. It's who you are. You have opened yourself to *what is* every step of the way.

N: I try. That's my goal.

RM: And now acknowledging missing the next 20 years?

N: The blessed Mary is a help in her acceptance of fate that cannot be changed. It's a very difficult fate. I can't imagine it. I taught medieval art history, and it's awash in glorified virgins, you know (chuckles). I've always wondered: What if somebody came at me and said, "Guess what? You're going to be pregnant by somebody. Nobody will believe you. No one will have any fun to start with, and it will not be like you had a rapturous night of love (chuckles). It will just be boom! Pregnant! And you won't have a husband, and you won't have an explanation for things, and you won't have a life." (Chuckles.) Would you be giddy with joy? I don't think so. Her "yes" continues to be instructional to me. I'm trying to say "yes" to my life as it is now. I'm talking too much.

RM: And you're talking about a "yes" to your fate as well.

N: Oh, yes. I'm talking too much. I need my air. I need you to talk.

RM: That's because I've got too many questions, but I'm just going to make some observations and then see if you want to comment on them. You're managing your heart, your feelings, and the mechanics and logistics well—body changes, a new bed. You are more energetic, even in sadness. The energy is in your voice and spirit. I notice that you are picking up a little more fluid, I think, which might affect your walking.

N: Yes, I have to be really careful when I walk. I've started dabbling a little in Ativan for dealing with anxiety and a kind of shaky quiveryness. Ativan really knocks me out.

RM: It can relax you and should help quiet your thoughts if you have intense fear or panic.

N: That's what I've been using it for—the fear.

RM: You're doing a great job of juggling the medicines, bathroom, and bed—all the changes—and working with many different people as well as confronting fear and sadness.

N: Thank you. I am learning to manage the way other people affect me. That was part of the Sally-learning—putting up fences and encouraging people not to telephone because my natural disposition is to want to include everybody, relate to everyone, and accommodate everyone. I just don't have the strength. I adore Anna above all. She's the gentlest person, and when she came today at 5:15, for the first time ever, I said, "Dick McQuellon is coming at 6, and I think I need to rest a little before he comes." That was very hard. I'm sure she was glad to be told, but for me, it was a real departure. That experience with Sally was salutary. I haven't let her in so close to me again. She's here; she's daughterly, affectionate, and helpful—in some ways, indispensable. It was easy to let her have too much access to me. We are much too different for that to happen. So I'm learning.

RM: You are wise to continue with your "cocooning" and your retreat from some people. There is a rhythm about this, about how you let whom in, when, and what energy comes to you and from whom at different times. You are managing the people part of this well. You've come a long way.

N: (Chuckles.) *We* have come a long way!

Commentary: The interpersonal dimension in cancer care and especially at the end of life can be difficult. Closing out relationships with dear friends at the end while becoming increasingly dependent on new professionals, strangers admitted by necessity, is hard. They have direct access like no other people, even spouses, largely due to the patient's physical needs and emotional state. Such intense dependency can heighten vulnerability.

Nell requires help with the basic activities of daily living, such as eating, bathing, and walking. In her interaction with Sally, whom she loves dearly, she feels her vulnerability acutely. She wants to limit Sally's access to her because their spiritual worlds differ radically. Nell hopes to avoid conflict in her peaceful home cocoon.

RM: You've got your hospice people trained, too!

N: They are doing better. I want to know what other questions you have.

RM: You are doing well with mechanics as well as the transcendent, with prayer and a routine with Al at the end of the day. I can imagine the beauty of the music at night as you put yourself to sleep by tending to your heart, head, and spirit in prayer with your partner.

N: Yes, it is comforting. I do have occasions of sleep apnea, where I wake up for air. For the most part, my lungs are clear. I am sleeping beautifully. I usually get up twice to go to the bathroom and then go right back to sleep. Any other questions, good doctor?

RM: You're alive! I just want to remind you, it's OK to be alive. I think you've come around to that?

N: That's right, and I'm glad to be alive. I needed to learn it is OK. (Both chuckle.)

RM: I have some poems that I can read to you, and then we can bring Al in for closure.

N: Yes.

RM: This is by Ted Kooser, the poet laureate of the U.S. We discussed him a couple of weeks ago. This first poem is from *Delights and Shadows*.[9] (Box 11.2).

RM: A glimpse of the eternal—that's it.

N: That's the whole poem?

RM: "Just now, a sparrow lighted on a pine bough right outside my bedroom window, and a puff of yellow pollen flew away." Yep, that's it. Isn't that an interesting title, "A Glimpse of the Eternal"?

N: Wonderful. It's a *koan*.

RM: Yes, a bit of a riddle. This next one by Kooser is titled "A Happy Birthday." (Box 11.3)

N: Wonderful. Good stuff. Yes!!

RM: These Kooser poems seem suited to you with your love of nature, birds, and the landscape. He is a keen observer of the natural world, as are you.

N: Thank you. There was a beautiful rain storm this afternoon.

RM: The trees are full with the nourishing rain. It's peaceful here now. (Al enters the room.) Hello, Al. Nell was just telling me about the wonderful custom you have at night with prayer.

A: Yes, we pray together. It means a lot to us.

RM: I will let you be for your prayer time and take my leave now.

Box 11.2 A Glimpse of the Eternal

Ted Kooser

Just now,
a sparrow lighted
on a pine bough
right outside
my bedroom window
and a puff
of yellow pollen
flew away.

Final Commentary: I chose the Kooser poems because of their simplicity and depth. Nell has taught me about glimpsing the eternal with her observations about nature. The eternal can be seen in the moment, each moment. It is all we have—one moment following

Box 11.3 A Happy Birthday

Ted Kooser

This evening, I sat by an open window
and read till the light was gone and the book
was no more than a part of the darkness.
I could easily have switched on a lamp,
but I wanted to ride this day down into night,
to sit alone and smooth the unreadable page
with the pale gray ghost of my hand.

another. Nell is beginning to "ride this day down into night." Her last night is moving closer. I can see it coming.

Al escorts me to the door this night; we are close, bumping shoulders as we walk. He beckons to me with what he does not say. I feel the tug of his silence. Can he sense the end is near, and does he find some solace in my presence? He thanks me again for my wife Cyndee's visit. Since I was out of town, she delivered books by Frederick Buechner and Anthony De Mello to Nell. Al apologizes for not speaking with her longer. He is gracious and courageous in the face of Nell's progressive disease. Our talks have encouraged Nell to seek more emotional expression from Al. Even while Alzheimer's has slowed his thinking, he has found the ability to express tenderness and love for Nell, something that has been difficult for him. Nell feared her decline would tax him. He has remained steadfast, by her side, solid. Al invites me to have pizza with them. I decline, but now I have regrets about not staying. It was one of Nell's last meals. The old question returns, "Could I not do more?"

Notes

1. We had previously discussed Buber's version of an answer to the statement, "I am completely without hope." Smith, RG., *Martin Buber. Makers of Contemporary Theology*, (1967) Richmond, VA: John Knox Press, p. 14–15.

   One afternoon, after a morning of mystical contemplation, I had a visit from a young man I had never met, without being there in spirit. I certainly did not fail to let the meeting be friendly, I did not treat him with any less courtesy than his fellow students who were in the habit of seeking me out about that time of day for consultation and conversation. I talked openly and attentively with him, but I failed to guess the questions that he did not put into words. Later, not long after, I learned from one of his friends—he himself was no longer alive—what the essential content of his question was. I learned that he had come not casually, but borne by destiny, not for a chat but for a decision. He had come to me; he had come in this hour. What do we expect when we are in despair and yet turn to another person? Surely, a presence by means of which we are told that nevertheless there is meaning. Since then I have given up the "religious" which is nothing but the exception, extraction, exaltation, ecstasy; or it has given me up. I possess nothing but the everyday out of which I am never taken. The mystery is no longer disclosed, it has escaped or it has made its dwelling here, where everything happens as it happens. I know no fullness but each mortal hour's fullness of claim and responsibility.

2. Roethke, T. (1975). *The collected poems*. Garden City, NY: Doubleday. See Box 8.2 in Chapter 8.
3. The concept of the bodhisattva is central to the Mahayana Buddhist tradition. A bodhisattva is someone who seeks enlightenment both personally and for others and is primarily characterized by compassion, an empathic sharing of the sufferings of others.
4. Rinpoche, S. (1992). *Tibetan book of living and dying*. New York: Harper Collins.
5. Tonglen reverses the usual human logic of avoiding suffering and seeking pleasure. Someone practicing it visualizes taking in another's pain with every in-breath and sending out a specific benefit on the out-breath. The process helps to liberate meditators from old patterns of selfishness and to begin to feel love for, and to take care of, others and themselves.
6. Wilbur, K. (1991). *Grace and grit: Spirituality and healing in the life and death of Treya Killam Wilber*. Boston: Shambala Press.
7. Beuchner, F. (1992). *Listening to your life: Daily meditations*. New York: Harper Collins.
8. De Mello, A. (1982). *The song of the bird*. New York: Doubleday.
9. Kooser, T. (2004). *Delights and shadows*. Port Townsend, WA: Copper Canyon Press.

12

June 14, 2005—Facing, Accepting and Yielding

Before you know what kindness really is
you must lose things,
feel the future dissolve in a moment
like salt in a weakened broth.
What you held in your hand,
which you counted and carefully saved,
all this must go so you know
how desolate the landscape can be
between the regions of kindness.

Nye, N. S. (1984). Kindness. In *Words under the words: Selected poems* (p. 42). Portland, OR: Eighth Mountain Press.

Main Themes: Our dialogue as a process; experiencing the kindness of caregivers; facing death while getting an uncooperative cable TV to work, an unusual conundrum.

Nell greets me at the door tonight—a first. She immediately excuses herself, walking gingerly on swollen feet and calves to the restroom. She is thin, fading. Therese Schroeder-Sheker has described cancer patients as "disappearing slowly." In an earlier conversation, Nell joked that she was disappearing like Tinker Bell, a fairy who, in some versions of J. M. Barrie's play *Peter Pan*, is portrayed as a fading light revived by audience applause.

Nell's humor is reserved tonight. She walks cautiously to the living room, nasal cannula in place, oxygen tube trailing, and asks me, "Would you like a Coke?"

"Yes," I say.

I watch her move slowly and deliberately to get two Diet Cokes from the pantry. She opens one can and places a straw in it. For me, she wrestles with the ice-cube tray, runs water over it, trying to loosen the ice. I can see it is a great labor and want to give her a hand, but hesitate. She smiles, places six ice cubes in the glass, and says, "That's as far as I go, sir."

I follow her to her room holding the oxygen tube and her drink. She sits on the bed, winded, thankful to be seated. As she adjusts herself, I walk back to the kitchen, pick up my soda, and comment to Al, "You're good, but she's very good!" He nods, smiles. He usually gives me a glass of water when we meet. Nell has assumed his role tonight and served up a welcome shot of caffeine after a long day. What a gift to be in the midst of this couple—Al, stable and dependable as a rock; Nell, moving gracefully toward the end, if a bit wobbly right now.

Nell is a brave woman. She is grateful for the kind people in her life. She believes that kindness will come to her aid as she moves through to the end. She has expressed gratitude since our very first meeting.

Dialogue 12

RM: You were saying that you view our conversation as a developmental sequence?

N: Yes. As I go farther into the illness, I learn things. I have to learn them well before I learn new things. I think they build on one another. I've gone back to Dialogue 4 and read straight through sequentially, so I can bring out the bones of whatever I think will help other people. We don't arrive at cut-and-dried positions on things and then check them off our list of developmental tasks. I keep learning and then needing to learn more in the end.

RM: I agree.

Commentary: In Chapter 6, Nell named the developmental sequence she is experiencing: face death, accept it, and yield to it. This process has been dynamic and a recurring theme throughout our time together. She is now yielding.

N: As my body becomes weak and helpless and stuck in bed, in a finite state, I seem to be developing an enhanced capacity to understand the process. This journey was bigger than the nightgowns! (Laughs.)

Commentary: In Chapter 8, Nell discussed her struggle over purchasing two expensive nightgowns even as death approached. She feared they would arrive and she would be gone. Her conflict recalls the warning, "Don't buy green bananas Who knows if you will be around to eat them?"

RM: And that is big!

N: We know the nightgowns were very big! Then we bought a new TV, and I could not get it hooked up. Failure to get it working, just crept into my mind and took over. I woke up in the morning with this feeling of dread. I had followed the directions for 60 minutes on how to use the TV. I understood what Al was doing. I also understood what he didn't understand what he was doing. (Chuckles.) He really couldn't help me beyond getting me back to the large signal. I was pretty sure that if I called Time Warner up and said, "Would you send somebody out to fix this?" they would say, "It's not our problem because it's a DVD/VCR problem, and we just take care of the box." I stewed about this Saturday. It was a day of total fatigue, really pressing fatigue, and I didn't call anybody. Al read a lovely Thich Nhat Hanh story[1] to me, and I read some haiku and just refreshed myself on the basics of getting things into proportion and how much—how out of proportion—I can get. I was out of proportion on getting this TV set up and working!

Commentary: Before I could ask her to tell me more about the developmental sequence of learning, Nell spoke about the frustration of cable TV setup, something I can relate to. TV is a diversion that helps her turn down the constant background buzz of death. She can be mindful even while feeling irritated by a television that will not cooperate. Her frustration with the TV mirrors her struggle with other obstacles to yielding to death on the near horizon.

RM: Reading Thich Nhat Hanh is very good for helping get back perspective.

N: Yes. I made myself a vow that Sunday I would not even try to turn on the TV. Thich Nhat Hanh says elsewhere in a wonderful book on mindfulness that it is very important to take one day a week that is not available for all this stuff, a day when you don't allow these irritants in. I did that Sunday, just paying attention to the moments. You devote your day to centering and cleaning your reflective self. I had a wonderful professor in college, a really productive scholar, and yet on Sunday, he never ever cracked a book. Saturday afternoon he listened to the opera. Sunday he did church and his prayers and meditation, and then he would go to the arboretum or go for a walk or visit friends. He was very disciplined in setting time aside.

RM: I like that.

N: I have realized how difficult it is to get to that discipline. I remembered my professor's discipline and Thich Nhat Hanh's ideas, and I thought, "This day I will set aside for self-care, being mindful, and I will not touch this machine!!"

RM: Great. Did it work?

N: It worked on Sunday. Monday, I knew I had to do something. I still was very, very tired. I didn't wake up until late. Lori comes at 12:30, so by the time I'd showered, there wasn't time to tackle the TV. I must have awakened at 11. There wasn't time for an hour of tech support conversation, so I presented all of this to her because she has been reading some of my Thich Nhat Hanh books with great appreciation. She likes them and knew his work already. She's read a biography of the Buddha with Thich Nhat Hanh and a number of really good books. I knew she would understand both dimensions of this. I was laughing and saying I just feel that this is what all the meditation is about, to get you to a place where you could handle this kind of absurd stress.

RM: I'm with you.

N: Jack Kornfield wrote a book called *After the Ecstasy, the Laundry*.[2] You still have to come back to doing laundry. In my case, after facing death, I come back to getting this damn TV working! I asked Lori if she knew anyone who might be smart with setting up cable TV. She said one of her male people—her son or husband—could help. I was thrilled!

Commentary: *Nell observes that we are learning along the way and then illustrates a conundrum with her television. I was surprised by her abrupt transition from reflection on her psychological development to the TV problems.*

After the Ecstasy, the Laundry *illustrates the idea that we cannot escape the mundane in favor of contemplating the transcendent. The ordinary tasks of daily living hold our lives together. Still, considering mortality is heavy work. In* The Unbearable Lightness of Being, *Milan Kundera contrasts a life where nothing matters (actions are light) to a life where everything matters (actions are heavy).[3] Nell's reflection suggests that she moves between light and heavy.*

RM: Now you have consultants!

N: She was so on-the-spot. They were here at 5 p.m. Monday, and we had a sweet visit. Oh, they're such nice people. They got the

TV all fixed up, and it works like a charm. I'm not scared of it, and I know who to call if it starts talking back to me. (Laughs.)

RM: That's great.

N: Well, it was. It's like watching the moles in your garden. They're underground, and you can't see them, but you can see their effects. It was rather like that—my underground catastrophe. Not only is it working, Dick, but here's the real payoff. I then called Time Warner to see what it would cost to add the Tennis Channel. And thinking that they would probably say, like, $4.95 or something that, I would probably say, "Oh, it's not worth it." She said 95 cents a month!

RM: So now you've got tennis anytime you want?

N: It's nonstop. I left it on mute today, just had it as a background, just for the joy that it was here. They have archives—you have got to fill the airwaves with tennis! They have our tribal material, old film, Wimbledon, Bjorn Borg—oh, just marvelous.

RM: Bjorn Borg had some real matches, didn't he?

N: Yes, yes, he did!

Commentary: *Tennis is a passion of Nell's and one way for her to escape intrusive thoughts of dying.*

RM: Can we talk about how you're feeling?

N: Yes. I feel better, except my stomach aches, and my legs are tired, but I got a fair amount of time up today, and I did a lot of editing here in the bed, which now I have to plug into the screen. I'm feeling pretty good.

RM: I read what you sent me. You are making our conversation more precise as well as illustrating important points. Just the point you made earlier—realizing there's a progression, there's a development here—that isn't apparent in one single conversation.

N: Yes, that's right. I mostly cut out a lot of verbiage and try to make the points a little clearer.

RM: OK. One of my concerns has been that recording and reading the transcript would take energy from you. It seems OK?

N: It's really giving energy to me! And many wonderful things have happened. This wonderful thing—creep week—it just crept up on me.

RM: Creep week?

N: Yes, how things creep up. Pat came twice and massaged my legs really from the groin to the toes; she just eased some of that edema. And Dr. T increased the medications, and the combination of the two drugs—a water pill and the other—has given me better balance. I'm not steady on my feet at all—very, very unsteady—but better than I was. I gave our dear friend Bill my last piece of antique furniture that was in the other room so that we can move the wheelchair out of Al's way. It won't be an impediment for him. I'm trying to streamline the apartment to simplify and to keep my mobility as long as I can.

RM: You're doing great: the massage, and the increased Lasix [a medication to prevent fluid retention], and the other medication Dr. T is giving you help lessen the discomfort when you bend the legs.

N: Bending at all had pretty much gone, so it's much, much better. The trouble is sitting up. The edema pulls at my legs when I sit up. It pulls and aches, and then it's time to go back to bed, and so I have to just gauge it and follow my body, listen to my body.

RM: Well, you're doing a fine job of gauging, listening to your body, and maintaining your joy even with discomfort. I see joy in your face—your eyes and your smile.

N: The good thing is so many kind people. I was talking to Al yesterday about the kindness that comes into our lives. Lori comes; Bill comes and takes Al to lunch; and Anna comes and brings me the paper. All so kind to me. Audrey's coming tomorrow, and I told her that I would like an assessment of mobility because you told me to. So there! (Smiles and laughs.)

RM: All right, good work. (Chuckles.)

N: I want to stay home, to be able to stay here. I'm highly motivated that way.

RM: It's reasonable for you to stay home.

Commentary: Nell wants to die at home. She does not want to be "shipped to hospice," as she puts it, unless absolutely necessary. Fortunately, she has an excellent medical oncologist who has managed her pain medication, even as hospice assumed some in-home care. Nell has remained clearheaded and able to take her medications as needed. Her ability to manage her medical/physical needs as well as to contemplate death is remarkable, especially considering she has only eight days to live.

N: Yes. And I think that my energy is a kindness, too. Naturally, it is wonderful to have some sense of value and purpose with our conversations, and I enjoy working with words.

RM: You have value and purpose without reading and editing our conversations. And you feel additional value and purpose as you do this work?

N: Yes. We both want it to happen.

RM: I agree. Now, let me backtrack just a bit. You said you want to stay home, and you are motivated to stay home. Tell me more about that.

N: Well, just managing incontinence is a problem. I'm working on it. I'm working on various combinations of Depends underwear and so forth. Sharon is a less steady helper than I had hoped she would be, so I probably need more help. We've talked about this. We will be looking at adding some other help because we are seeing things like changing the water on the humidifier—now that's a trick for me to get down there.

RM: Good thinking. The oxygen is working fine, right?

N: It's fine. I didn't tell you, but one night I changed it, and I thought it was secure, but it wasn't, and no oxygen would come out, so fortunately, I didn't panic; I called the supplier, and she identified the problem right away. She said it happens all the time. But there will be a time when I will need someone to come in every day for things like changing that stuff. We're just going to go ahead and arrange for that now.

RM: OK, good.

N: I have the name taped to the door. It's the name of the woman at Bayada nursing who should come do an assessment. So I'm thinking about more help here.

RM: Are you ready for more help this week?

N: No. I do see it coming soon. I'll see what Audrey says tomorrow. I was hoping she would tell me where hospice stops. I'm going to talk to her tomorrow.

RM: So someone is here with you when you need them. You've been great with managing hospice care, finding some flexibility with hospice, too, because they don't usually cover transfusions, and yet you had one!

N: That was Dr. T who got that, obviously.

RM: You're managing a lot well. You're not seeking additional help too soon nor waiting to the last minute. Your timing is good. I know timing has been a concern of yours all along.

N: Thank you, yes. Because of what we're doing, our writing, I am begging my body to hang on. I want to do this, and I think my body wants to do this, too, so I think you've got me for a while. (Laughs.)

RM: Well, of course, our project will never be whole without a reader.

Commentary: *What I meant was that the dynamic process of writing and editing can only be completed by readers. I am afraid Nell thought I meant that her time would run out before our project could be completed. As it turned out, she would not read all of our transcribed conversations before her time ran out. We are on borrowed time now, a reality we cannot see this night, a reality I want to avoid.*

N: I don't suppose it will [be completed] since I'm only on tape four. My realization is that the tumor is an independent entity. It is on its own level, calling the shots. At some level, I have no bewitching powers over the tumor.

RM: We can't bewitch the tumor, but you have been managing the changes in your body—the edema, the pain, the growth of the tumor, and all that comes with it. At the same time, you are staying close to the trees, the sky, the sun, and the breeze through the window.

N: And the wonderful prayer time and listening to *Rosa Mystica*. Ending the day with that is just lovely. It is so beautiful. Al and I listen to it every night together.

RM: What a wonderful end to the day! I sent an email to Therese Schroeder-Sheker, telling her how much you appreciate the music. Your appreciation is known to the producer.

N: I would love to read the piece, the article that she wrote. Could you hand me my case? The type is very small. There, footnote 4—she apparently did an article that was included in a book called *Maps of Flesh and Light*, edited by Ulrike Wiethaus of Wake Forest.[4] I would love to get ahold of that chapter, very, very much.

RM: I will get it for you.

N: I know the book is out. I've seen the book a couple of years ago, and I think what would be really wonderful is if you could get an offprint of that article.

RM: Sure. "The Use of Plucked Stringed Instruments in Medieval Christian Mysticism." I will get it. I see you are nodding off now. I will leave you and Al to your nightly ritual.

N: Thank you, I am sleepy.

Commentary: We end somewhat abruptly, as Nell's eyes slowly droop. She is weary. Even though she speaks of having good energy, I can see the changes in her body and recognize she is failing. Greeting me standing at the door tonight, serving me the drink, must have taken great effort. Did she know this recorded session would be our last? As I walked to my car, I could not admit to myself the end was so near.

Notes

1. Hanh, T. N. (2002). *No death, no fear: Comforting wisdom for life.* New York: Riverhead Books. A passage in the section titled "Waves are Water" (p. 23) provides comfort: "When you look at the surface of the ocean, you can see waves coming up and going down . . . Looking deeply, we can also see that the waves are at the same time water. . . . A wave may say, 'I have been born and I have to die' . . . But if the wave bends down and touches her true nature she will realize that she is water. Then her fear and complexes will disappear."
2. Kornfield, J. (2000). *After the ecstasy, the laundry: How the heart grows wise on the spiritual path.* New York: Bantam Books.
3. Kundera, M. (1984). *The unbearable lightness of being.* New York: Harper and Row.
4. Wiethaus, U. (1993). *Maps of flesh and light: The religious experience of medieval women mystics.* Syracuse: Syracuse University Press.

13

June 21–22, 2005—Departure

You cannot go into the room where someone is dying and not pay attention. Everything is pulling you into the moment. And for me it is one of the most alive places to be. It's an extraordinary gift.

> Ostaseski, F. (2004). Living and dying each day. In
> V. J. Dimidjian (Ed.), *Journeying east: Conversations on aging and dying* (p. 27). Berkeley: Parallax Press.

June 21, 2005

Nell's ending has begun. First, she phoned me.

N: I feel like I'm in free fall. The energy has dropped out of the bottom. I feel terrible. Can you find out if insurance pays for a transfusion?

RM: I will do my best to find out who knows the answer to that question. I'll talk with you tonight when I get that information.

N: Can you do better than that? I don't know if I can come out of this.

RM: Yes, I will try.

A low-energy alarm went off in Nell today. She called in distress at 2:30 p.m. Just seven days ago, she stood, walked, and served me a Diet Coke. Now she can hardly raise her head off the pillow and is desperate for help.

"Can you do better than that?" I wonder how I can be useful here—how I can do "better than that." The nagging question remains: Can I not do more?

I page Nell's physician. We talk about her situation, about what she seeks, about the cost of healthcare, about what is "indicated." Dr. T tells me a transfusion is not indicated in this situation. I trust his judgment, yet I wonder why not? Is Nell's request unreasonable? Why can't I do something—help her with just one more transfusion? Is that too much to ask?

Nell felt this way just three weeks ago on May 30, and a transfusion gave her energy and new life. She craves energy now, as she is profoundly lethargic. She tells me she wants to complete our project. I tell her again our project is whole but will be fully realized only when readers enter our story through these conversations. It is my duty to ensure that happens.

I bring the transfusion question to my colleagues in a staff meeting. I ask them what they might do, how I might pursue it. Would you push for another hospital visit, knowing the many challenges it would present? We talk about the ethical pillars of care: "first do no harm" and "do some good." How do they apply here? Would attempting a transfusion do more harm than good given Nell's physical status and the logistics of transportation to a medical facility? Would her insurance company refuse to cover the cost? In any case, without a doctor's order, a transfusion is impossible. Perhaps we are discussing a moot point. We achieve no clinical consensus.

When I arrive for our scheduled appointment that evening, I see intense worry on Al's normally impassive face. As I step into Nell's room, I understand why. She is withered, disappearing before my eyes. In just one week, she has changed dramatically. Her swollen abdomen has shrunk. Her skin and eyes look yellow—her liver is failing. She does not ask to "go on record," to tape our conversation, as she normally would.

Even though she looks extremely frail, she pulls herself up in the bed and asks me to move some furniture and objects in her bedroom to make it easier for Al to walk about. She points out several objects she wants to give to me. We settle in for our talk. Her gaze is steady. She tells me she feels too weak to attempt a transfusion and has made peace with her decision to give over to the call of death. She woke to the pecking of cardinals at the feeders this morning but has slept much of the day. She is now actively dying—facing it, accepting it, and yielding to it gracefully, just as she had hoped. She thanks me for hearing her story, for recording and preserving her life in mortal time, for the gift of this transition period. Nell has discovered the healing power in telling her story of forgiveness and the renewal of important family relationships.[1] Al sits quietly, acknowledging Nell's words. He speaks occasionally, resigned to what this day brings.

Her voice is quiet and soft, her eyes occasionally closing for short periods when she appears to be summoning the strength to speak. She is at peace here. She has been searching for this place for much of her adult life. She found it in the company of her husband, their household, and our conversations. I have been privileged to share this time with her, to walk with her toward home. I recall the passage she sent me from *My Ántonia*.[2] Just like Ántonia, Nell looks as if she is sitting in a garden, leaning against a pumpkin, sun shining on her smiling face. She is becoming part of something larger, something entire, whether it is sun and air or love and goodness. It is coming as naturally as sleep. She is nearly home.

I can feel Nell leaving, the bond of our relationship dissolving. In my professional career, I have never walked so closely with a person actively contemplating and reflecting on her own death. This is true ambivalence, my heart holding on, my head letting go, simultaneously. I don't quite know what to make of having been so close for so many weeks and now watching her go.

Nell has arrived at the threshold she has been seeking for months. Her body is weak, but her spirit is strong and prepared. She is ready, letting go. Rather than sinking into deep mourning or talking about disappointment or sadness, we share stories from Nell's life. I realize I may never see her alive again. I want to banish this thought, which has intruded on me often over the course of our time together, but it is persistent. I do not think that I am communing with her spirit for the last time. Why do our meetings, our conversations in mortal time, give me hope?

Nell smiles as she speaks of tennis and the Wimbledon tournament this summer. A spark of energy ignites her tired eyes. She is alive. I hold her hand as we speak, now looking into those steady eyes that are ready to yield. I place my hand on hers and Al's over mine. We hold hands in prayer and in silence. I bend over to kiss Nell on the cheek, squeeze her hand. Her eyes close, and she smiles. I feel her grip on my hand loosen, and I draw away.

Al walks me to the door. He whispers, "Thank you," as I walk out. I am ambivalent—sad and grateful, tearful yet celebrating that Nell's peaceful ending is so near. I want to return to the comfort of my own family tonight, but I'm moving slowly. I'm heavy with sadness yet thankful that Nell has suffered so little in these last days. I don't know where to go. I don't know what to do with myself.

I walk down the long halls of Creekside Terrace Apartments. Purple carpet with green diamond shapes, simple paintings on the walls, light-colored ash doors with silver handles and locks, the sound of a vacuum cleaner, the clink of silverware and dishes below as the dining area is cleaned. I walked these halls to 13 meetings. I did not expect so many. Meetings with Nell became conversations that heal with Nell and in the end, Al. We did not record tonight.

I am carrying a box with gifts from Nell and Al: two teacups by a potter named Duff; a beautiful bowl crafted by a man whose name I cannot remember; *Master Potter* by Shoji Hamada[3]; *The Essential Haiku: Versions of Basho, Buson, and Issa,* edited by Robert Haas[4]; *Bring Me the Rhinoceros: And Other Zen Koans to Bring You Joy* by

John Tarrant.[5] In that one, Nell told me to start with number 10, "The great way is not difficult." We began our story with a quote from Seng-ts'an: "The great way is not difficult if you just don't pick and choose."[6] Our journey is ending with me holding Nell's treasures. She entrusts them to me.

A gentle rain falls as I make my way to the car. A faint rainbow appears in the east. I see green merging into yellow and red. I cannot see its end, high in the sky.

As the rain trickles and stops, the sun pokes out of the gray clouds as it slides away into this night. I look again for the rainbow. It's gone. You are almost home, dear Nell.

June 22, 2005

Al calls late in the day. I leave the office and hurry to Creekside Terrace Apartments. He ushers me to Nell's room, saying only, "I think she is leaving us."

We sit at the bedside. Nell's eyes at half-mast are glassy. Her mouth is slightly open, and she breathes deliberately, only occasionally struggling for air. She is wearing one of the beautiful nightgowns she bought online, fearful she might die before they arrived, leaving Al with an unpleasant costly surprise. Her hair is combed and pulled back neatly, arms by her side, hands bluish and cool. I reach to hold her hand. Is that a slight squeeze I feel? Did the corners of her mouth move up ever so slightly? Does she know I am here? I lean over and whisper, "We did it, Nell. Our story is complete. You are leaving a gift of love in this world. Thank you." I turn to see Al with his sad smile. We sit together, waiting. How long will we sit? How long will Nell hover near bardo, the state of existence between death and rebirth, according to some schools of Buddhism?

We wait in silence. A gentle breeze moves the sheer curtains. A cardinal lands on her birdfeeder, turns toward us, stares. Pecks at the seed. Stops. Is she listening? Nell grimaces three times and then emits a barely audible, high-pitched sound. No death rattle or struggle like I have seen. I watch the pulse in her carotid artery, clearly standing out from her thin neck. It has been beating steady. Now it slows and stops. I wait for it to return, one more beat. Nothing.

We wait for 10 minutes. Will her heart beat one more time? Only yesterday, we talked here of wholeness, our project, our conversation in mortal time. I thanked her for her generosity and courage in sharing her story with me. I thanked her for the gift of her trust, for allowing me into her heart, home, and family. I told her she has shown me a way to walk gracefully in the deepening shade of illness.

I turn toward Al and say, "She's gone." He nods. I'm not sure he understands. I put my arm around him and feel him tremble. I want to say something comforting, but no words come. We watch Nell in silence for some time. Is she really gone?

Her hospice nurse Sally sits quietly in the next room. I ask her to join us in prayer. She enters and immediately launches into a loud, God-seeking prayer, assuming I had invited her to lead. For some reason, I cannot ask her to stop, so I can "pick and choose" our prayer, to paraphrase the *koan* that Nell liked so much. This seems a fitting end, one Nell would have found amusing. Even with two guardians at her side, she gets a send-off that none of us would have anticipated or chosen. As Nell taught, all we need to find enlightenment is to accept that we can't "pick and choose" our path. What I wanted was not to be, yet what happened was fitting if a bit zealous for Nell's taste. She would laugh at this last wrinkle in mortal time, evidence of a God with an ironic sense of humor. We had talked of plans and what might happen as the end approached. I noted that my grandmother often repeated the old saying, "Man proposes, God disposes." We are all sailors, hauling up canvas, seeking the wind, following it best we can to our hoped-for destination, the beginning of another great adventure.

You made it home, Nell. I saw you depart and hope you find your dream of unconditional love waiting in the next world.

Notes

1. See McQuellon, R. P., & Hurt, G. J. (1993). The healing power of cancer stories: A book review essay. *Journal of Psychosocial Oncology, 11*(4), 95–108.
2. See Chapter 7, Box 7.1; Cather, W. (1918; 1994). *My Ántonia* (p. 20). New York: Penguin Books.
3. Hamada, S., Wilcox, T., & Kikuchi, Y. (1998). *Shoji Hamada: Master potter.* London: Lund Humphries Publishers, Ltd.
4. Haas, R. (Ed. and Trans.). (1995). *The essential haiku: Versions of Basho, Buson, and Issa.* New York: Ecco Press.
5. Tarrant, J. (2004). *Bring me the rhinoceros: And other Zen koans to bring you joy.* Nevada City, CA: Harmony Books.
6. Seng- ts'an. (2014). *Hsin- hsin Ming: Verses on the faith-mind* (R. B. Clarke, Trans.). http:// www.mendosa.com/ way.html

14

Afterword—Therapist Reflections

A witness assures us that our stories are heard, contained, and transcend time.[1]

All shall be well, and all shall be well and all manner of thing shall be well.[2]

Julian of Norwich

Nell's death was peaceful—just what she had hoped for all these months and what we had worked toward for weeks. Al and I were her witnesses. We watched her last heartbeat in those final moments. I had never been so close to death. I drove slowly back to my office, grateful and sad, and stayed there until later in the day. My patients were waiting. The reality of this calling: One person dies; another steps up. Every day, a parade of people enters the kingdom of suffering and healing. Some are filled with grace; others are sunk in their discouraging reality, perhaps overwhelmed by tenacious physical symptoms, changing relationships, intrusive thoughts, and feelings of sadness, depression, and anxiety. Who will find healing? Who will be lost? What makes the difference?

For Nell, it was her intention to embrace and learn from her dying. Even as she withdrew from her wide web of relationships, she expanded her interior world of possibility and prepared for her immense journey, her transition to infinity. She was alive to her disease process, curious about it, and able to articulate her feelings directly, with humor and wonder.

From our first meeting, she was drawn to the concept of mortal time and its application to her life. We had both read *Tuesdays with Morrie* in which Mitch Albom, a former student, relates Professor Morrie Schwartz's philosophical reflections on coping with amyotrophic lateral sclerosis (ALS), a progressive disease that eventually leaves its victims helpless and unable to move.[3] Like Morrie, Nell was open to exploring her philosophy and feelings as metastatic breast cancer pushed her toward the end.

Her reflections on living in mortal time are the core of this book. We recorded our conversations because we believed we could inform patients and caregivers who were on the same path, but I had reservations: Would recording change our interaction and render counseling less useful to Nell? Would we be self-conscious about the process, preoccupied with finding "the right words," inhibiting our spontaneity? Could our conversations be woven into a coherent story? These questions faded as we both benefited from our rich dialogue and insights that might one day benefit others.

Nell shared her vibrant life with her friends and family. She saw the connections among all things and found peace and comfort in nature, especially what she saw from her window—the line of maples and oaks in the woods; cardinals, finches, Carolina chickadees at the feeders; glowing sunsets and the breeze that stirred the curtains next to her deathbed. The moon rising, her lunar beacon.

Nell's beloved cat Amber was a constant source of security. He provided touch comfort—what Nell called "tactility"—when he snuggled in the bed with her. His presence became increasingly important as she weakened. She would reflexively stroke him when she spoke with me, and he purred with regal satisfaction, condescending to her love from his lofty perch.

She opened her life to me and in doing so, made peace with the ragged edges in her story that had been carved over the years. We completed the work of forgiveness and repair, not knowing in the beginning that this would be the result of our dialogues.

To paraphrase philosopher Hans Gadamer, a real conversation is never the one we wanted to create.[4]

Cultivating Self-Knowledge by Witnessing

According to Aristotle, knowing oneself is the beginning of all wisdom. Reading these transcripts helps me to see who I am as a therapist. I see our relationship emerge out of our interactions. I considered my responses and opportunities to respond differently. It did not occur to me that one day I would scrutinize my own work when reviewing the transcripts. My initial reaction was negative: What was I thinking when I said that? Many times during our meetings, I searched for the right words or chose the silence of "being with" as the most useful response. My contribution to Nell's words was listening to her narrative. She was teaching me about living, dying, and letting go in a way I had not known.

The great death in my life had been my father's. He died suddenly at age 46 of a massive heart attack on the eve of my parents' 25th wedding anniversary. I was 21 and more than 3,000 miles away in Seattle while he died in my mother's arms in Nassau, Bahamas. I will always remember our family doctor's words: "Richard, your father died of a heart attack last night." His words penetrated, sending me into shock, deep weeping anguish. I flew home to Peoria, Illinois, blinded by grief.

Encounters with patients who are dealing with life-threatening illness call for humility. Reading these dialogues does indeed humble me. With time and absorbing colleagues' responses to the transcripts, I am less critical and more accepting of my limitations. Whatever mistakes I made in our conversation, whatever pathways we could have traveled but did not, the therapeutic relationship we developed was transformative.

I thought I knew and understood Nell's illness narrative because we lived it together. However, in editing these dialogues and listening carefully to her voice again, new meaning has emerged. It's as if I am witnessing a second story, hearing our conversation in a new key, entering it as the observing narrator. Talking with Nell helped me to understand mortal time lived out in the shadow of metastatic breast cancer.

Suffering, sadness, grief, anger are feelings any caregiver may contend with during these precious end-of-life moments. How can a therapist manage the emotional pull when the loss/death of the relationship is the inevitable outcome? I felt the impending loss acutely while learning more about Nell's life. We grew closer. She lived values I hold dear—an appreciation for nature and the connection of all creation, the importance of family, friendship, and conversation; the possibility after death that she named "unconditional love," reverence and a search for a loving God waiting on the other side. The great sadness that came over me in the last days of her life contended with our celebration of achievement. There was little comfort in our success at the time; it took months to develop. If I could convince myself that letting go of a life well lived was a success, my grief would be eased.

The Nell dialogues were and are a constant reminder of my own mortality, an invitation to consider my own hoped-for narrative. I would like to end like Nell, with a few adjustments to the script. How many times have I been speaking with a patient suffering from a debilitating, disfiguring cancer and thought, "That could be my story". My father's sudden death gave me a possible narrative that I have accepted since 1970, updating it over the years. Is it my fate to drop dead suddenly and unexpectedly of a massive heart attack, as he did? Will one of the two leading causes of death in the United States, heart disease and cancer, be my companion in the end? Or maybe an accident? Now another grim possibility—SARS-CoV-2. I look at the projected number of pandemic deaths and wonder if I might be among those statistics one day. Is this trepidation an occupational hazard for any professional caregiver working in mortal time, considering best and worst endings? I hope it is not a morbid preoccupation with death but rather a reminder of mortality and a motivation to see possibility in each moment. I feel this positive spark most in the company of my grandchildren. Their presence is a source of laughter, hope, and energy. In their company, I am alive to each moment.

Therapist as Bodhisattva

I am grateful for Nell's kind reference to me as a bodhisattva, a special compliment. I think of my calling as a "guide in Cancerland," sometimes leading all the way to the end, as with Nell. An image of Guanyin, the Buddhist bodhisattva of compassion, drawn by my colleague, Gail Hurt, RN, MA, hangs over my office desk. Guanyin was first given the title "Goddess of Mercy" by Jesuit missionaries in China. The Chinese name is short for Guanshiyin, which means *perceives the sounds of the world.* Gail's rendering of Guanyin is a reminder that expressing compassion and guiding patients and caregivers at our comprehensive cancer center are a sacred vocation and my duty.

Guanyin is generally thought to derive from the Sanskrit Avalokitesvara, a male form; early representations of bodhisattvas were always masculine, while later images might show female and male attributes. According to the Lotus Sutra, bodhisattvas can magically transform their bodies as necessary to relieve the suffering of others, so Guanyin is neither woman nor man. As an enlightened one, the bodhisattva is free to dwell in nirvana but instead remains in life to comfort and guide others to nirvana. In Mahayana Buddhism, to which Chinese Buddhism belongs, gender is no obstacle to enlightenment. The Bodhisattva Kuan Shih Yin travels the world in a variety of shapes, conveying beings to salvation.

In the end, I sat with Nell as she passed into the next world, to her salvation.

"The Mummers'
Dance": Grief-Evoking Sounds

"The Mummers' Dance" by Loreena McKennitt was my elixir late Tuesday nights after meeting with Nell when the house was quiet. I would block the outside world with the noise-canceling headphones and hear the haunting melody but not the words as my tears would flow—for Nell and for the hundreds of patients I had known over many years as a professional caregiver. This grieving ritual helped me to return to cancer medicine, freed and cleansed for the moment. It is ironic that the Celtic tradition of mumming referenced in this song released my grief. Mumming is a cultural practice primarily associated with springtime, fertility, life, but it helped me to grieve the slow, visible loss of Nell.

When leaving her bedside, Nell would ask me to turn on her CD player so she could listen to Teresa Schroeder-Sheker's soothing *Rosa Mystica*. It pulled at my grief, a grief that still pulsates regularly, stimulated by my daily encounter with sad stories, made bearable by the company of trusted others. When in need of uplift, I would play the song "My Healing" from the album *God Is Still Doing Great Things* by the interracial choir Shades of Praise. It's inspirational, and it rocks.

The Eulogy: Roots and Ambivalence

Spirituality meant a great deal to Nell, and her faith became more important as her death approached. She drew on her Catholic Christian beliefs while incorporating Buddhist concepts, attempting to reconcile her ambivalence about the church as institution in contrast with the church as her people. Reading through the transcripts clarified how prominent her beliefs were in our conversations. We shared the same Catholic faith tradition and belonged to the same parish. I knew the priests and volunteers who visited her regularly and was able to facilitate those meetings.

Nell asked me to give her eulogy, a great honor and a welcome burden. With her family and friends in attendance, I told our story, describing Nell's courage in mortal time. She was brave enough to reveal her thoughts and feelings while facing down her imminent death. I quoted the poem she wrote about the space we shared in my office, where mortality was no longer the elephant in the room but a welcome conversational partner. I spoke of Nell's many accomplishments, her doctorate in art history, her editing work with Studs Terkel, her love of art, and her many teaching positions, from university level to middle school. Her most cherished role and achievement was teaching eighth-grade language arts and social studies at the Hill Magnet School for the Performing and Visual Arts.

I concluded with a phrase Nell often used: "The great way is not difficult if you just don't pick and choose." Nell opened herself to her fate, not picking and choosing so much, but facing, accepting, and finally, gracefully, yielding to death. We did not move on to the cemetery, as Nell chose cremation. This church service was my ritual letting go, the end.

What Legacy Did Nell Leave for Her Therapist and Readers?

How long can any legacy last? One generation? Who pays attention to history, even their own family history? The dying can be obsessed about what to leave their loved ones: a last letter, a recording, an object? Some enterprising entrepreneurs have proposed leaving a video on the gravestone. Would it help those remaining?

My sojourn in mortal time leads me to believe that the effects of love and kindness flow down through the generations, whether their sources are consciously remembered or not. These qualities can take root in the hearts of those touched by them and bloom as they are passed on. We leave our love and a bit of ourselves in the spirit of those who remain. We live on through acts of loving-kindness.

In the poem "Turning Point," Rainer Maria Rilke writes, "For looking, you see, has a limit. And the more looked-at world wants to be nourished by love. Work of seeing is done, now practice heart-work upon those images captive within you."[5] Images remain in me, from conversations in mortal time with Nell and hundreds of other patients over these years. As I leave the day to day conversation in mortal time, the work of seeing patients and hearing their stories is ending. What does it mean to practice heart-work with those images? It means remembering my mortal time companions with compassion. They dwell in me with undertonesof sorrow and hope. To embrace these images with respect and gratitude is to live in the spirit of the bodhisattva.

Notes

1. Pikiewicz, K. (2013, December 3). The power and strength of bearing witness. *Psychology Today*. https://www.psychologytoday.com/us/blog/meaningful-you/201312/the-power-and-strength-bearing-witness/
2. Starr, M. (2013), Showings of Julian of Norwich: A New Translation. Kindle edition (p.67) Charlottesville: Hampton Roads Publishing, Inc.
3. Albom, M. (1997). *Tuesdays with Morrie: An old man, a young man, and life's greatest lesson*. New York: Doubleday.
4. Gadamer, H. G. (1989). *Truth and method* (p. 385). London: Sheed and Ward.
5. Rilke, R. M. (2003). Turning point. In *Turning-point: Miscellaneous poems, 1912–1926, selected and translated by Michael Hamburger* (p. 53). London: Anvil Press Poetry.

Index

Boxes are indicated by *b* following the page number